Global Health Programs and Partnerships

Evidence of Mutual Benefit and Equity

AUTHORS

Jonathan A. Muir
Jessica Farley
Allison Osterman
Stephen E. Hawes
Keith Martin
J. Stephen Morrison
King K. Holmes

A Report of the CSIS Global Health Policy Center and the University of Washington Global Health START Center, in collaboration with the Consortium of Universities for Global Health

March 2016

CSIS | CENTER FOR STRATEGIC & INTERNATIONAL STUDIES

START CENTER

Consortium of Universities for Global Health

ROWMAN & LITTLEFIELD

Lanham • Boulder • New York • London

About CSIS

For over 50 years, the Center for Strategic and International Studies (CSIS) has worked to develop solutions to the world's greatest policy challenges. Today, CSIS scholars are providing strategic insights and bipartisan policy solutions to help decisionmakers chart a course toward a better world.

CSIS is a nonprofit organization headquartered in Washington, D.C. The Center's 220 full-time staff and large network of affiliated scholars conduct research and analysis and develop policy initiatives that look into the future and anticipate change.

Founded at the height of the Cold War by David M. Abshire and Admiral Arleigh Burke, CSIS was dedicated to finding ways to sustain American prominence and prosperity as a force for good in the world. Since 1962, CSIS has become one of the world's preeminent international institutions focused on defense and security; regional stability; and transnational challenges ranging from energy and climate to global health and economic integration.

Thomas J. Pritzker was named chairman of the CSIS Board of Trustees in November 2015. Former U.S. deputy secretary of defense John J. Hamre has served as the Center's president and chief executive officer since 2000.

CSIS does not take specific policy positions; accordingly, all views expressed herein should be understood to be solely those of the author(s).

ISBN: 978-1-4422-5908-9 (pb); 978-1-4422-5909-6 (eBook)

Center for Strategic & International Studies
1616 Rhode Island Avenue, NW
Washington, DC 20036
202-887-0200 | www.csis.org

Rowman & Littlefield
4501 Forbes Boulevard
Lanham, MD 20706
301-459-3366 | www.rowman.com

Contents

Executive Summary

Academic global health programs are proliferating and global health partnerships between North American academic institutions and institutions in low- and middle-income countries (LMICs) are steadily increasing. This study employs surveys and key informant interviews to examine global health partnerships and presents a framework for success to guide the development of sustainable global health programs and partnerships with measurable, defined impact.

Eighty-two North American academic institutions and 44 international partnering institutions participated in the survey. Key informant interviews were conducted with global health leaders at 15 North American academic institutions and 11 partnering international institutions. Quantitative data were analyzed using linear regression, and qualitative data were used in thematic analyses.

The surveys and interviews provide evidence of mutual benefits resulting from these global health partnerships as well as areas for further development and improvement. Key conclusions include:

- Overall, there was near unanimous agreement between North American academic and international partnering institutions that global health partnerships are beneficial. North American institutions are somewhat more positive than their international partners in their assessments of certain benefits, both for themselves and for their international partners.
- Greatest impact in perceived benefits is seen for education and research collaborations, but favorable benefits were reported by most partners across all additional areas of global health partnerships examined (e.g., maximizing global health impact, leadership development, training and mentoring, and health systems strengthening).
- Some inequities are perceived in global health partnerships, specifically in terms of decisionmaking (related to the one-sided provision of funding), in the lack of bidirectional student exchange, and sometimes in publication authorship.
- Students are a great resource and source of energy in North American global health programs, but their needs and expectations must be managed. Moreover, perceptions varied regarding the adequacy of North American student training and preparation, with cultural awareness and language training emerging as key areas of

concern. Common suggestions for increasing student preparation include placing more emphasis on training to introduce students to the culture and customs of their destination countries before arrival, bolstering language training when feasible, and increasing the awareness of visiting students of the challenges and limitations of working in low-resource settings.

- The demographic composition of global health partnerships is in flux, with both international institutions and North American academic institutions looking forward to diversifying their partnerships. While the vast majority (97 percent) of international institutions cited South-North collaborations as the most valuable to date, nearly 40 percent say that developing South-South collaborations will be their highest priority in the future. Similarly, many North American academic institutions are expanding their networks of affiliation to partner with other North American and European academic institutions.
- The most common strategy described by global health leaders at North American academic institutions for establishing their own programs was to unite existing global health partnerships and projects established by faculty members on campus. The implicit intra-institutional goals for these North American institutions have been to create synergies and to marshal interdisciplinary expertise; to increase efficiency and avoid duplication internally as well as externally with international partners; to develop new institutional global policies, guidelines, and standards; and to gain influence.
- Funding is critical, but not the only factor in program success. While institutional financial support was emphasized the most, institutional and faculty leadership support, personal relationships, global health champions, student enthusiasm, effective communication, and time for partnerships to mature were all highlighted as important factors.

This study represents partnerships and programs from just over 80 percent of member institutions of the Consortium of Universities for Global Health (CUGH) as of 2015 and from 67.7 percent of the members of the Association of American Universities. For CUGH members, we hope that this study will contribute to a better understanding of global health partnerships as mutually beneficial collaborations and offer points to consider for institutions seeking to establish, maintain, or improve their global health partnerships and programs. However, we anticipate that the relevance of these findings can and should extend beyond the current CUGH membership. In its 2013 Global Health Programs Database, CUGH listed 157 North American academic institutions with global health programs. However, in the United States alone there are over 2,900 postsecondary Title IV institutions granting four-year degrees and some offering masters or doctoral degrees. With this in mind, there is the potential that global health programs and international partnerships may continue to proliferate across North America and in low- and middle-income countries, and thereby come to broaden the scope and global impact of many of these institutions and their partner institutions. These future opportunities will be highly dependent on the continuing flow of funding. Given the preliminary evidence presented in this study suggesting that global health programs and partnerships are realizing positive mutual benefits, we encourage funding organizations—for example, the Gates Foundation, the Clinton Foundation, the Canadian International Development Agency (CIDA), the International Development Research Centre (IDRC), the National Institutes of Health (NIH), the United States Agency for International Development (USAID), and UN agencies—and academic institutions themselves to further their support of these programs and partnerships.

Introduction

In May 2014, the Strategic Analysis, Research, and Training (START) Center of the Department of Global Health at the University of Washington (UW), in collaboration with the Center for Strategic and International Studies (CSIS) and the Consortium of Universities for Global Health (CUGH) reported on the *Sustainability and Growth of University Global Health Programs*.[1] That report used data collected from online surveys and key informant interviews to explore the tremendous growth of global health at U.S. universities, the variations in size and scope of programs, core competencies associated with global health, training for students, funding, and leadership. The challenges of defining and achieving mutually beneficial partnerships with international institutions were not specifically examined.

Questions around definition, assessment, and mutual benefits of international partnerships are the focus of this follow-up study. Effectiveness of collaborations between partners was assessed in terms of the mutual development of goals; collaborative planning, implementation, and evaluation of performance; and mutual benefits. The rapidly growing interest in global health education and training, research, and service at universities has led to a surge in international partnerships. These partnerships stand to benefit from a timely assessment of how well the partnerships are working and how they can be improved to maximize synergy and mutual benefits.

The process of developing and sustaining partnerships, specifically between North American academic institutions and institutions in low- and middle-income countries, merits greater exploration. The University of Washington, in collaboration with CSIS and CUGH, conducted this follow-up study to appraise whether and how international partnerships are mutually beneficial to both North American academic institutions and their international institution partners. The study assessed determinants of equity, benefit, harm, and sustainability of partnerships, as well as the emerging global health impact of these partnerships.

This study had two objectives:

1. Examine the mutual benefit of international partnerships in global health programs at academic institutions, including determinants of equity, benefit, harm, and sustainability.

1. A. I. Matheson, J. L. Walson, J. Pfeiffer, and K. Holmes, "Sustainability and Growth of University Global Health Programs," Center for Strategic and International Studies (2014).

2. Develop a strategic roadmap to guide North American academic institution global health programs and their international institution partners in developing sustainable collaborations, with measurable and defined impact.

Background

That academic global health programs are proliferating is beyond dispute.[2, 3, 4] According to CUGH estimates, in 2011 there were 78 North American schools with a "comprehensive" global health program, defined in part as having at least one partnership with an institution in the Global South, up from six schools in 2001.[5] Global health programming at North American academic institutions continues to grow; over 100 North American academic institutions are now members of the Consortium of Universities for Global Health, which listed 157 North American academic institutions with global health programs in its 2013 Global Health Programs Database. Global health partnerships between North American academic institutions and institutions in low- and middle-income countries have increased as well. Many of these partnerships developed "organically," often building on the international connections of an individual North American faculty member.[6] Not all partnerships have formal or sustainable funding mechanisms, and the functions of these international partnerships vary, from collaborative research to hosting students from partnering institutions. In some instances there has been limited oversight in how these partnerships function and no standardized measurement of impact.[7]

Traditional global health partnership models often involve financial flow from North to South, with goals and priorities set primarily by the financing institution. This has raised concerns "about the one-sided nature of those relationships that limit partners in low-resource areas from setting the agenda or benefiting from outcomes."[8] Alternative models have recently been explored. The Medical Education Partnership Initiative (MEPI) began as a five-year (2010–2015), President's Emergency Plan for AIDS Relief (PEPFAR)-funded initiative that distributed funding to principal investigators (PIs) at 13 institutions in sub-Saharan Africa and allowed them to then distribute funds to their North American partners.[9] The MEPI initiative has recently been partially renewed, with $35 million committed to training junior faculty in eight African countries in the next five-year phase.[10] Another model was piloted by the University of Michigan and its partners in

2. J. P. Koplan et al., "Towards a Common Definition of Global Health," *Lancet* 373, no. 9679 (2009): 1993–1995.
3. R. Beaglehole and R. Bonita, "What Is Global Health?," *Glob Health Action* 3 (2010): 5142.
4. M. Rowson et al., "Conceptualising Global Health: Theoretical Issues and Their Relevance for Teaching," *Globalization and Health* 8, no. 36 (2012): 2–8.
5. M. Merson, "University Engagement in Global Health," *New England Journal of Medicine* 370, no.18 (2014): 1676–1678.
6. Ibid.
7. M. Morse, "Responsible Global Health Engagement: A Road Map to Equity for Academic Partnerships," *Journal of Graduate Medical Education* 6, no. 2 (2014): 347–348.
8. E. O. Olapade-Olaopa et al., "Growing Partnerships: Leveraging the Power of Collaboration Through the Medical Education Partnership Initiative," *Academic Medicine* 89, no. 8 (2014): S19–S23.
9. Ibid.
10. NIH, "NIH Commits $36M to Train Junior Faculty in Africa," *NIH News and Events* (2015): 1.

Ghana (including academic institutions and the Ministry of Health) who met in Ghana and developed a charter for collaboration that established principles to guide their partnership. The charter was adopted and signed by all participants,[11] continues to inform this partnership six years later, and has subsequently informed the process of establishing new global health partnerships at the University of Michigan. However, these commendable efforts have yet to be more widely adopted by North American academic institutions.

Further understanding is needed of how international partnerships function, from both the North American and international institution perspectives. The present study has two objectives: first, to evaluate to what extent these partnerships have been mutually developed and are mutually beneficial, and to identify determinants of equity, benefit, harm, and sustainability. Second, we aim to use these findings to suggest processes, considerations, and best practices to guide North American and international institutions as they engage in global health programs and partnerships.

Methods

We employed a mixed methods assessment of North American academic institutions and their partnering international institutions engaged in global health. We conducted surveys and key informant interviews sampled from leaders at these institutions. We anticipated that our two objectives would be highly related and thus opted to approach these two objectives synergistically in our research methods. We also undertook a literature review to inform suggestions for processes, considerations, and best practices to guide development of global health partnerships.

SURVEYS

The quantitative component of our mixed methods approach comprised two web-based surveys: one for North American academic institutions with global health programs (for this study, "academic institution" encompasses universities, colleges, and schools of higher education, as well as centers within these institutions) and one for international partner institutions identified by North American survey respondents. Both surveys were developed as part of an iterative process and were first vetted by representatives of both North American and international institutions. The surveys included a combination of semi-quantitative questions, often in the form of Likert scales, and open-ended questions that allowed for more subjective answers. Appendix A and B provide copies of the two survey instruments.

CUGH member institutions located in North America were identified through the CUGH membership list. Non-CUGH institutions were identified through a CUGH database on all known North American global health programs,[12] cross-referenced with former CUGH

---

11. F. Anderson et al., "Creating a Charter of Collaboration for International University Partnerships: The Elmina Declaration for Human Resources for Health," *Academic Medicine* 89, no. 8 (2014): 1125–1132.

12. "2013 Global Health Programs Database," Consortium of Universities for Global Health, http://cugh.org/resources/2013-global-health-programs-database.

membership lists. Ultimately, 121 North American institutions (101 CUGH members and 20 non-CUGH members) were identified. While we recognize that many strong global health programs exist at academic institutions throughout Europe, they were outside the scope of our research and were not included. The surveys were disseminated by research assistants in the UW START Team and facilitated by the office of the Executive Director of CUGH. Overall, global health leaders from 85 institutions responded to the survey, including 82 (81.2 percent) of the 101 CUGH member institutions and three (15 percent) of the non-CUGH institutions (see Appendix D). Given the low response rate among non-CUGH institutions, we restricted our analyses to the CUGH members. Among respondents, 46.5 percent directed the global health entity at their institution; 16.3 percent were chancellors, deans, chairpersons, or held other leadership positions; 16.3 percent were program administrators; and the remaining 20.9 percent were faculty professors.

North American survey respondents were asked to identify up to three international partner institutions—one high-performing partnership, one middle-standing partnership, and one struggling partnership. Using the contact information gathered from these responses, we distributed surveys to 62 international partner institutions identified in North American surveys. Forty-seven international partners from 44 different institutions undertook and returned surveys. Respondents represented different programs at the three institutions that had two respondents and in all three cases these institutions were partnered with different North American academic institutions. The North American online survey, which contained 30 questions, was conducted from May 18 to October 15, 2015, and the 43-item international partner survey from June 8 to October 15, 2015.

Original dissemination of both surveys was accomplished through an online survey tool.[13] An electronic (Microsoft Word) version was later disseminated to help increase response rates from respondents who struggled with the online survey format.

Survey data formally incorporated into this study were first cleaned and analyzed using Stata.[14] Descriptive statistics are defined and then depicted in figures throughout this report, but the statistical analyses used to assess our qualitative findings require additional explanation of the variables involved.

Dependent Variables

North American Academic Institution (NAAI) Self Benefits is a composite scale that combines the ratings from Question 19 in the survey of North American academic institutions. This question asks respondents to rate the extent to which they perceive international partnerships as beneficial for their global health program in seven categories (i.e., student/trainee knowledge acquisition; attracting prospective students, trainees, and faculty; collaborative research; building student foundations for careers oriented toward global health; developing leadership; diversification of revenue for the North American academic

13. Survey Gismo, http://www.surveygizmo.com/.
14. StataCorp LT, *Stata Statistical Software* (Release 11) (College Station, TX: StataCorp LP, 2009).

institution; and maximizing global health impact). The ratings of benefit were organized as Likert scales and recoded for analytic purposes so that 1 = Harmful, 2 = Not Beneficial, 3 = Somewhat Beneficial, 4 = Beneficial, 5 = Very Beneficial. Combining these ratings produced a variable with a potential minimum value of 7 and a potential maximum value of 35.

NAAI Benefits to Partners is a composite scale that combines the ratings from Question 22 in the North American Academic Institution survey. This question asks respondents to rate the extent to which they perceive their international partnerships are beneficial for international partners in eight areas (i.e., knowledge acquisition; financial support; collaborative research; training and mentoring; health systems strengthening; reciprocal student exchanges, education, and training; developing leadership; and beneficial local impact on health). The ratings were organized as a Likert scale and recoded for analytic purposes so that 1 = Harmful, 2 = Not Beneficial, 3 = Somewhat Beneficial, 4 = Beneficial, 5 = Very Beneficial. Combining these ratings produced a variable with a potential minimum value of 8 and a potential maximum value of 40.

International Partner Institution (IPI) Self Benefits is a composite scale that combines the ratings from Question 10 in the survey of international institutions. This question asks respondents to rate the extent to which they perceive their international partnerships are beneficial for their institution in nine areas (i.e., knowledge acquisition for students; knowledge acquisition for faculty and administrators; financial support; research support; health systems strengthening; interventions or services implementation support; technology and equipment transfer; reciprocal student exchanges; and maximizing global health impact). The ratings were organized as a Likert scale and recoded for analytic purposes so that 1 = Harmful, 2 = Not Beneficial, 3 = Somewhat Beneficial, 4 = Beneficial, 5 = Very Beneficial. Combining these ratings produced a variable with a potential minimum value of 9 and a potential maximum value of 45.

NAAI Collaborations is a composite scale that combines the ratings from Question 26 in the North American Academic Institution survey. This question asks respondents to rate how well their program is working together with its international partners in six areas (i.e., assessing the needs of their international partners; establishing mutual goals; addressing the needs of your international partners; planning, monitoring, and evaluating the impact of collaborations; soliciting and incorporating feedback from your students, faculty, and administrative leaders; and soliciting and assessing feedback from your university's international partners). The ratings were organized as a Likert scale and recoded for analytic purposes so that 1 = Not Done, 2 = Poor, 3 = Fair, 4 = Well, 5 = Very Well, 6 = Excellent. Combining these ratings produced a variable with a potential minimum value of 6 and a potential maximum value of 36. This dependent variable is used as part of the analysis investigating potential determinants of equity in global health partnerships. It is also used as an independent variable in some of the other analyses when the dependent variable came from the North American survey.

IPI Collaborations is a composite scale that combines the ratings from Question 18 in the International Institution survey. This question asks respondents to rate how well their program is working together with its North American partner academic institutions in five areas: assessing your institution's needs; establishing mutual goals; addressing the needs of your institution; planning, monitoring, and evaluating the impact of collaborations; and systematically providing feedback to your North American academic institution partners. The ratings were organized as a Likert scale and recoded for analytic purposes so that 1 = Not Done, 2 = Poor, 3 = Fair, 4 = Well, 5 = Very Well, 6 = Excellent. Combining these ratings produced a variable with a potential minimum value of 5 and a potential maximum value of 30. IPI Collaborations is also included in some of the other analyses as an independent variable when the dependent variable came from the International Institution survey.

IPI Needs Fulfillment is a composite scale that combines the ratings from Question 21 in the International Institution survey. This question asks respondents to rate how well their institution's needs are being met by their North American partners in seven areas: medical professional training program; collaborative research; clinical or public health interventions or services; health systems development/capacity building; technology exchange; policy development and advocacy; and learning and practicum experience for students. The ratings were organized as Likert scales and recoded for analytic purposes so that 1 = Not Done, 2 = Poor, 3 = Fair, 4 = Well, 5 = Very Well, 6 = Excellent. Combining these ratings produced a variable with a potential minimum value of 7 and a potential maximum value of 42.

Independent Variables

NAAI Funding Source is a composite scale that measures overall access to and importance of funding. Data come from Question 16 in the North American Academic Institution survey, which asks respondents to indicate the degree of importance of different sources of funding that are *currently received by their institutions* and *used to finance global health partnerships*. Potential funding sources include university funding, NIH funding (e.g., Fogarty grants, research grants), PEPFAR (HIV/AIDS related) funding, other federal government funding (e.g., CDC, USAID, etc.), nonfederal government/other external grants or contracts, private donor funding, and foundation funding. Rating of these sources were organized as Likert scales and recoded for analytic purposes so that 1 = Do Not Receive, 2 = Not Important, 3 = Low Importance, 4 = Medium Importance, 5 = High Importance, 6 = Essential. In addition, individual funding sources were analyzed as unique and separate independent variables. Combining these ratings produced a variable with a potential minimum value of 7 and a potential maximum value of 42.

NAAI NIH Funding Amount[15] is a continuous variable indicating the total dollar amount of NIH funding that a North American academic institution receives overall; this amount is not disaggregated to indicate amounts used to fund global health programs or partnerships.

15. NIH, "The Research Portfolio Online Reporting Tools (RePORT)" (2015).

NAAI Endowment[16] is a continuous variable indicating the total dollar amount of the institutional endowment at a given North American academic institution; this amount is not disaggregated to indicate amounts used to fund global health programs or partnerships.

NAAI—Private Institution is a dichotomous variable coded as Public = 0 and Private = 1.

NAAI—Part of Larger Institutional Partnership is a dichotomous variable coded as No = 0 and Yes = 1. This variable is included to indicate institutional resources available to NAAI global health partnerships due to incorporation into larger institutional-level partnerships. Data come from Question 13 in the North American Academic Institution survey, which asks respondents to indicate whether their global health partnerships are part of larger institutional or university partnerships.

NAAI Enrollment[17] is a continuous variable indicating the total student enrollment (both undergraduate and graduate) at a given North American academic institution.

NAAI Scope of Coursework, Certificate, Major, or Degree Offerings is a composite scale that measures the breadth of coursework, certificates, majors, or degrees offered by a North American academic institution. For a complete list of the individual offerings, please see Figure 2. Combining these ratings produced a variable with a potential minimum value of 7 and a potential maximum value of 13.

NAAI Assessment of North American Student Training is a composite scale that draws on data from Question 18 in the survey of North American academic institutions. Question 18 asks respondents to assess the degree of adequacy of the trainings or orientations provided to their students who participate in international global health partnerships. Potential training areas include ethics; host-country institutional requirements for visitors; sociocultural aspects of life in the host country; cultural awareness for engaging in international health work; language training; student's role, scope of tasks, and supervision while abroad; and preparation for the challenges of providing care or working in under-resourced settings. Rating of these sources were organized as Likert scales and recoded for analytic purposes so that 1 = Is Not Provided, 2 = Very Inadequate, 3 = Somewhat Inadequate, 4 = Somewhat Adequate, 5 = Adequate, 6 = Very Adequate. Combining these ratings produced a variable with a potential minimum value of 7 and a potential maximum value of 42.

IPI Funding Source is a composite scale that measures overall access to and importance of funding. Data come from Question 9 in the International Institution survey, which asks respondents to indicate the degree of importance of different sources of North

---

16. National Association of College and University Business Officers and Commonfund Institute, "U.S. and Canadian Institutions Listed by Fiscal Year (FY) 2014 Endowment Market Value and Change in Endowment Market Value from FY2013 to FY2014" (2015).

17. Data obtained from individual institutions' websites.

American funding that have been particularly critical for the success of their partnerships with North American academic institutions. Potential funding sources include North American academic partner(s); international research agencies (e.g., NIH, Fogarty International Center at NIH, Canadian IDRC); PEPFAR (HIV/AIDS related) funding; MEPI; other North American government funding (e.g., CDC, USAID, CIDA, etc.); nonfederal government/other external grants or contracts; UN agencies; international nongovernmental organizations (NGOs); private donors and/or philanthropy; and foundations (e.g., Gates, Rockefeller, Clinton). Ratings of these sources were organized as Likert scales and recoded for analytic purposes so that 1 = Do Not Receive, 2 = Not Important, 3 = Low Importance, 4 = Medium Importance, 5 = High Importance, 6 = Essential. Combining these ratings produced a variable with a potential minimum value of 7 and a potential maximum value of 66. In addition, individual funding sources were also analyzed as unique and separate independent variables.

IPI—Collaborations and Investments Received is a composite scale that draws on data from Question 12 in the International Institution survey, which asks respondents to indicate which of six types of collaborations or investments they receive from their North American partners. The International Institution survey provides a complete listing of the six types of collaborations or investments. Combining these ratings produced a variable with a potential minimum value of 0 and a potential maximum value of 6.

IPI Type of Institution is a categorical variable indicating whether an international institution is a public academic institution, private academic institution, NGO, government agency, or other. For analytic purposes, it is recoded as four dummy variables with Public Academic Institution serving as the reference category.

IPI Scope of Coursework, Certificate, Major, or Degree Offerings measures the breadth of coursework, certificates, majors, or degrees offered by an international academic institution. For a complete list of the individual offerings, please see Figure 6. Combining these ratings produced a variable with a potential minimum value of 0 and a potential maximum value of 13.

IPI Assessment of North American Student Preparation is a composite scale that draws on data from Question 16 in the International Institution survey, which asks respondents to assess the degree of adequacy of preparation of North American students hosted by their institution. Preparation areas of interest include ethical practices and host-country institutional requirements; sociocultural aspects of life in the host country; cultural awareness for engaging in health work in low- and middle-income countries; language training; understanding of role, scope of tasks, and supervision while in host country; and preparation for the challenges of providing care or working in under-resourced settings. Rating of these sources were organized as Likert scales and recoded for analytic purposes so that 1 = Is Not Provided, 2 = Very Inadequate, 3 = Somewhat Inadequate, 4 = Somewhat Adequate, 5 = Adequate, 6 = Very Adequate.

INTERVIEWS

To gain insights above and beyond the level of detail obtained in the two surveys, we interviewed 15 key informants working in global health programs at North American academic institutions, and 11 key informants at international partner institutions. Interviews took place between June 22 and October 27, 2015. Potential interview participants were identified from the completed surveys when a respondent indicated a willingness to be contacted for an interview. Interviews were carried out by phone, lasted approximately 30 to 45 minutes, and were conducted using semi-structured, open-ended interview guides (see Appendix C). Interview respondents were asked to briefly describe how their programs and partnerships were established and developed; assess the importance and/or benefit of these partnerships; define specific health goals being pursued through partnerships; identify challenges, successes, and areas for improvement; summarize lessons learned; and predict program/institutional sustainability. We documented interview responses using audio recordings and written notes. These notes were reviewed and coded to identify key themes and identify where differences arose among respondents. For lists of challenges, improvements, and recommendations provided by respondents, we grouped items thematically and recorded frequency of response type across all interviews.

LITERATURE REVIEW

To inform our strategic roadmap, we conducted a literature review to identify articles describing the establishment and development of North American global health programs. The search was conducted using PubMed and Boolean structured search terms. The 15 articles identified were then used as part of a cross-case comparison.

Survey Results

NORTH AMERICAN ACADEMIC INSTITUTIONS

Among the 82 North American academic institutions that participated in this study, 58.5 percent were public universities and 41.5 percent were private universities (Table 1). Across both public and private universities, 92.7 percent were from the United States, with a higher concentration located on the East Coast, and 7.3 percent of the North American academic institutions were from Canada. In addition, the North American academic institution participants represent approximately 67.7 percent of the Association of American Universities (AAU) university membership.

Of all respondent-reported global health entities (centers, institutes, etc.) 68.4 percent were a part of larger institutional or university partnerships (e.g., partnerships that operate beyond the institution's global health entity, are interdisciplinary, and include multiple global health programs). Over 80 percent operate at universities with over $10 million in NIH or Canadian Institutes of Health Research (CIHR) funding and over 90 percent are at universities with endowments exceeding $100 million. Figure 1 shows the geographic distribution of survey respondents.

North American academic institutions were asked to report on the number of programs and degrees that have "substantial global health components" that are offered by their institutions (Figure 2). Nearly all (94.9 percent) of North American academic institutions with global health programs offered at least one global health course. A Master of Public Health (MPH) or other health profession degrees (e.g., MD, RN, or DVM) with substantial global health components were also frequently reported, with over 50 percent of North American academic institutions offering such degrees. Certificates, postgraduate programs, or PhD programs with substantial global health components were also frequently reported.

Beyond the diverse educational programs and degrees with substantial global health content offered by the surveyed North American academic institutions, these institutions engage in a wide variety of other global partnerships, classified by the partnerships' content and activities (Figure 3). Overall, 93.5 percent of partnerships reported by North American academic institutions involved collaborative research, and 93.5 percent involved

Table 1. Characteristics of North American Academic Institutions Surveyed, n = 82

	n (%)
Public/Private	
Public	48 (58.5)
Private	34 (41.5)
Country	
United States	76 (92.7)
Canada	6 (7.3)
Part of Larger Academic Institutional Partnerships	
Yes	52 (68.4)
No	24 (31.6)
Overall (undergrad/grad) Enrollment (# of students)	
<2,500	7 (8.6)
2,500–9,999	11 (13.4)
10,000–40,000	48 (58.5)
>40,000	16 (19.5)
NIH/CIHR Academic Institution Funding* ($USD FY 2014)	
<10 million	14 (17.1)
10 million–49.9 million	22 (26.8)
50 million–200 million	27 (32.9)
>200 million	19 (23.2)
Endowment ($USD)	
<100 million	7 (8.8)
100 million–999.9 million	24 (30.0)
1 billion–5 billion	32 (40.0)
>5 billion	17 (21.2)
Association of American Universities (AAU)	
University Member	42 (67.7)

* National Institutes of Health (NIH); Canadian Institutes of Health Research (CIHR)

Figure 1. Locations of North American Academic Institution Survey Respondents

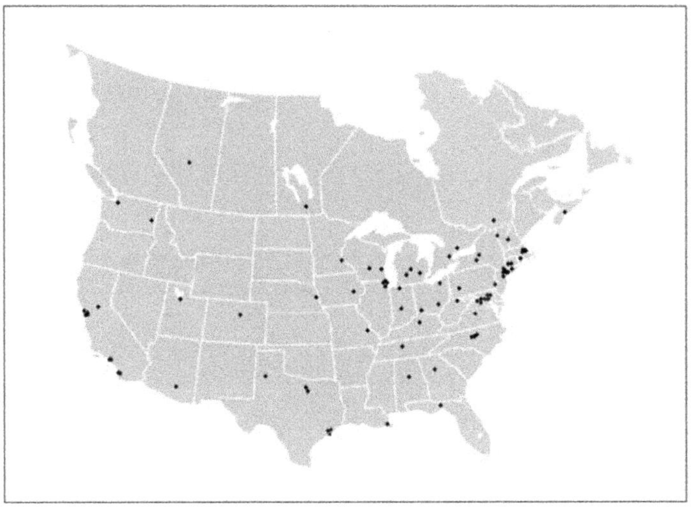

Figure 2. North American Academic Institutions' Coursework, Certificate, Major, or Degree Offerings with Substantial Global Health Components, n = 78

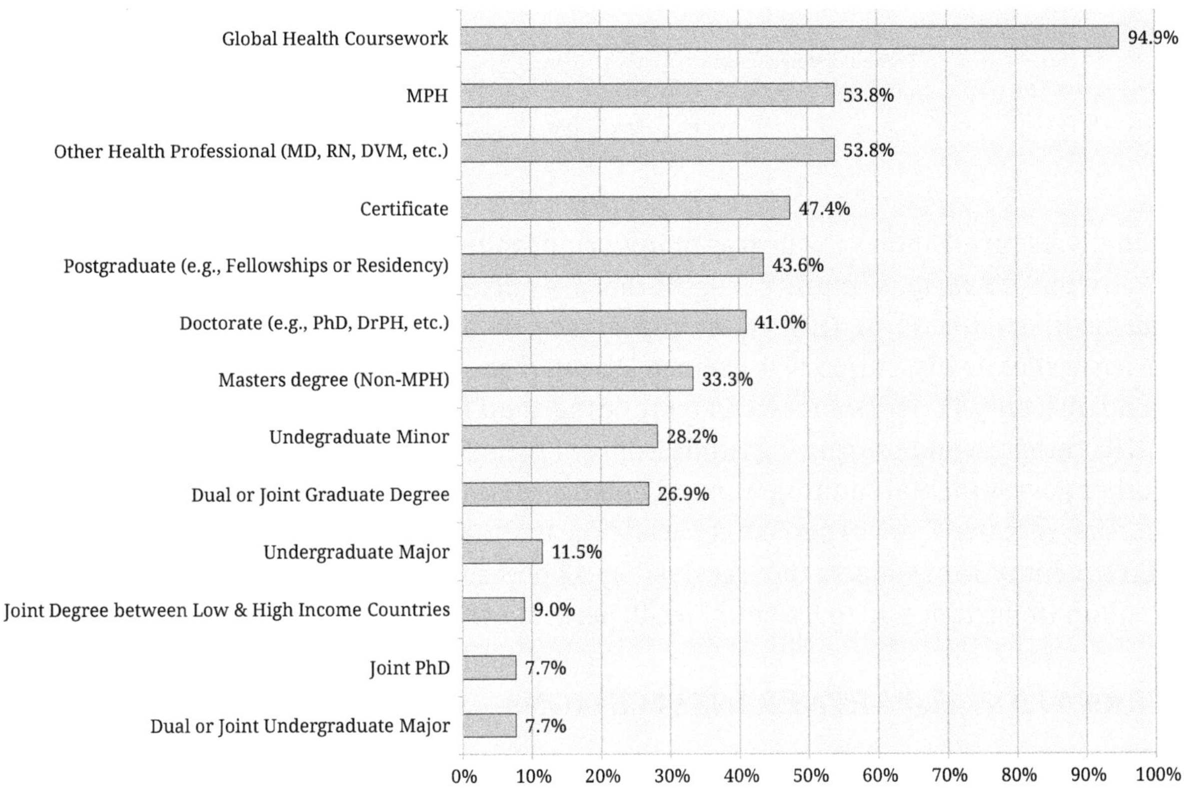

learning and practicum experiences for North American students. Of the four most common partnership types, three deal with some form of educational experience (e.g., student practicums, medical and health professional education, other health education). Partnerships focusing on health systems development, health interventions, policy development, and technology exchange were also frequently reported.

Figure 3. Types of Partnerships (North American Academic Institution Survey), n=77

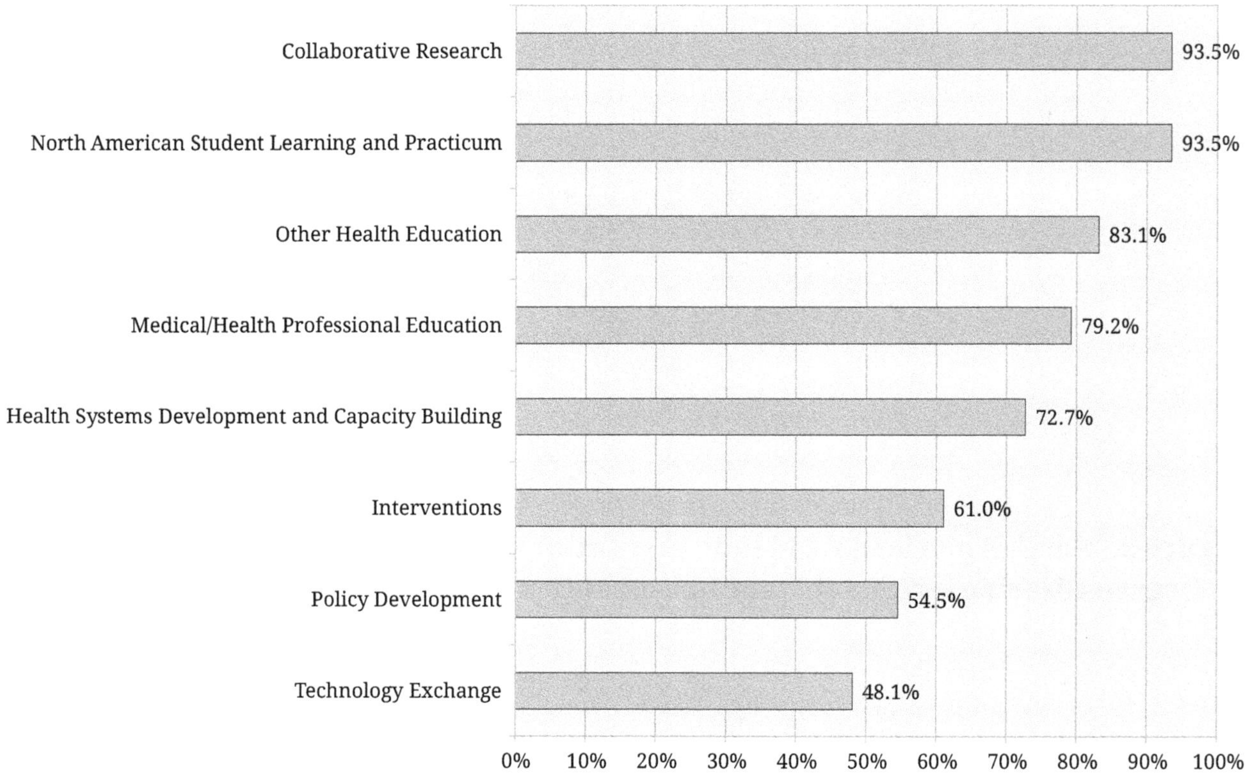

Finally, Figure 4 shows the degree of importance that North American academic institutions attribute to various funding sources that are currently received and used to finance global health partnerships. Of greatest importance, institutional funding from the North America academic institution was deemed *Essential* or of *High Importance* by 70 percent of respondents; only 11 percent received no funding at all from their own institution. Additionally, NIH research and/or training funds, support from foundations, private philanthropy, and other governmental funding were all noted as *Essential* or of *High Importance* by a large proportion (greater than 40 percent) of academic institutions. Interestingly, PEPFAR was the least frequent type of support (not received by 48 percent), but was nonetheless reported as of Medium Importance up to Essential by 40 percent of the North American institutions.

INTERNATIONAL PARTNER INSTITUTIONS

North American Academic Institution survey respondents identified 93 international partners (see Figure 5) and provided contact information for 62 of these partners. Some North American academic institutions actually also identified U.S.-based or high-income country partners (Spain, Germany); these were excluded from our analyses. E-mail invitations to complete the International Institution surveys were sent to those partners that were not excluded, and 48 (75.8 percent) responded (Appendix E). Of 47 international partner respondents, 72.3 percent represented public or private academic institutions, and 27.7 percent represented NGOs, governments, or other agencies (Table 2).

Figure 4. Importance of Various Funding Sources (North American Academic Institution Survey)

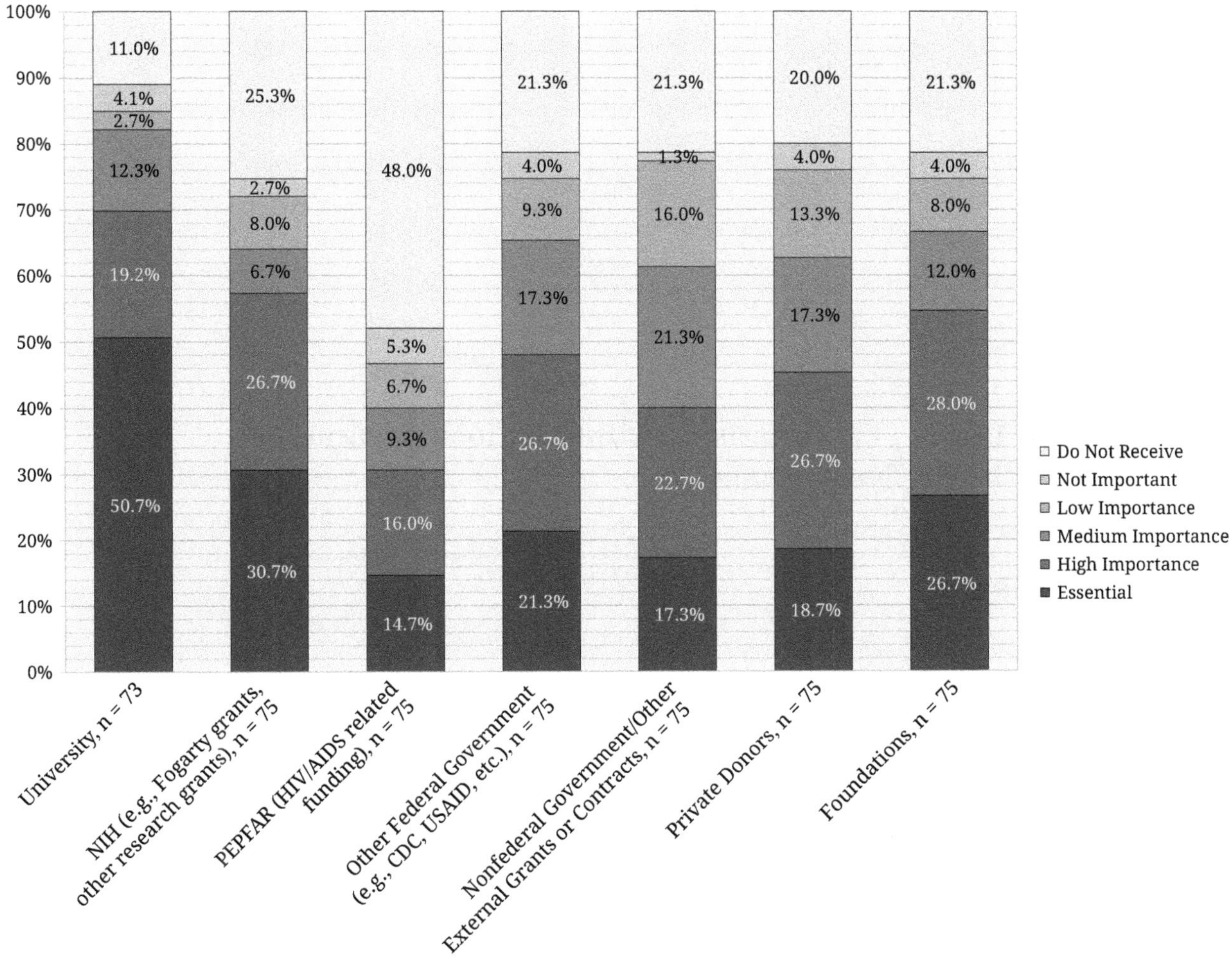

Respondents from the international institutions who completed the study survey identified a wide variety of focus areas (Table 2). More than half of these institutions indicated that they are engaged in health systems development and in HIV/AIDS and/or tuberculosis. Other common health-related focus areas include Maternal, Neonatal, and Child Health (MNCH); mental health; neglected tropical diseases; and chronic noncommunicable diseases and malaria. Health focus areas related to problems typically addressed by policy interventions, such as air pollution, tobacco and alcohol, traffic injuries, and violence, were less commonly reported. Moreover, a variety of other institutional foci (e.g., community education and empowerment, hygiene, ocean toxins, nutrition, and sanitation) were reported by fewer international partners.

International *academic* institutions reported on a variety of global health-related coursework, certificates, majors, and degrees offered by their institution, similar to the educational offerings of the North American academic institutions (see Figure 6 for a complete list of offerings). With one exception, all of the other types of education with substantial global health content were offered only half as frequently or less often by

Figure 5. International Partner Institutions Identified by North American Survey Respondents

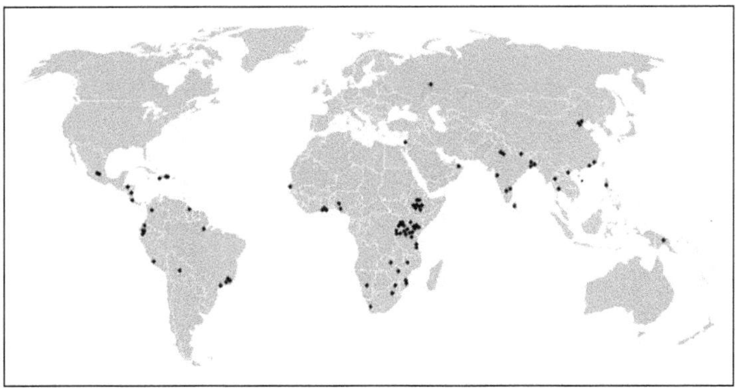

Table 2. Characteristics of International Institution Survey Respondents, n = 48

	n (%)
Region	
Africa	22 (45.8)
Asia Pacific	13 (27.1)
Latin America	13 (27.1)
Type of Institution	
Public Academic	29 (61.7)
Private Academic	5 (10.6)
NGO	9 (19.2)
Government or Other Agency	4 (8.6)
Areas of Focus of International Institutions (n = 28)	
Health Systems Development	20 (64.5)
Tuberculosis	20 (64.5)
AIDS/HIV	20 (64.5)
Maternal, Neonatal, and Child Health (MNCH)	16 (51.6)
Mental Health	15 (48.4)
Chronic Noncommunicable Diseases	13 (41.9)
Neglected Tropical Diseases	12 (38.7)
Malaria	11 (35.5)
Air Pollution	7 (22.6)
Road Traffic Injuries	7 (22.6)
Tobacco and Alcohol	7 (22.6)
Violence	5 (17.9)
Other	14 (45.2)

the international academic institutions as compared to North American academic institutions (as shown in Figure 2). The one exception was the joint degree, which was offered by just over 9 percent of the North American and 11.8 percent of the international academic institutions.

The numbers of partnerships reported by the international institutions are summarized in Table 3. Thirty-seven international institutions reported a total of 516 global partnerships. The number of such partnerships per international partner institution ranged from one to over 20, with the majority reporting six or more. Not surprisingly, the United States and Canada accounted for nearly half of global health partnerships reported by the international partner institutions surveyed in the study, which is to be expected given that the international institutions were identified by their North American partners.

Interestingly, however, even though these international partners were identified by North American institutions, just over 50 percent of all partnerships reported by the international partners surveyed were partners located in Europe, Asia and the Pacific, Africa, and Latin America (Figure 7). Clearly, the international institutions surveyed are actively engaged by a variety of global health partners from around the world.

Figure 6. International Academic Institutions' Coursework, Certificate, Major, or Degree Offerings with Substantial Global Health Components, n=34

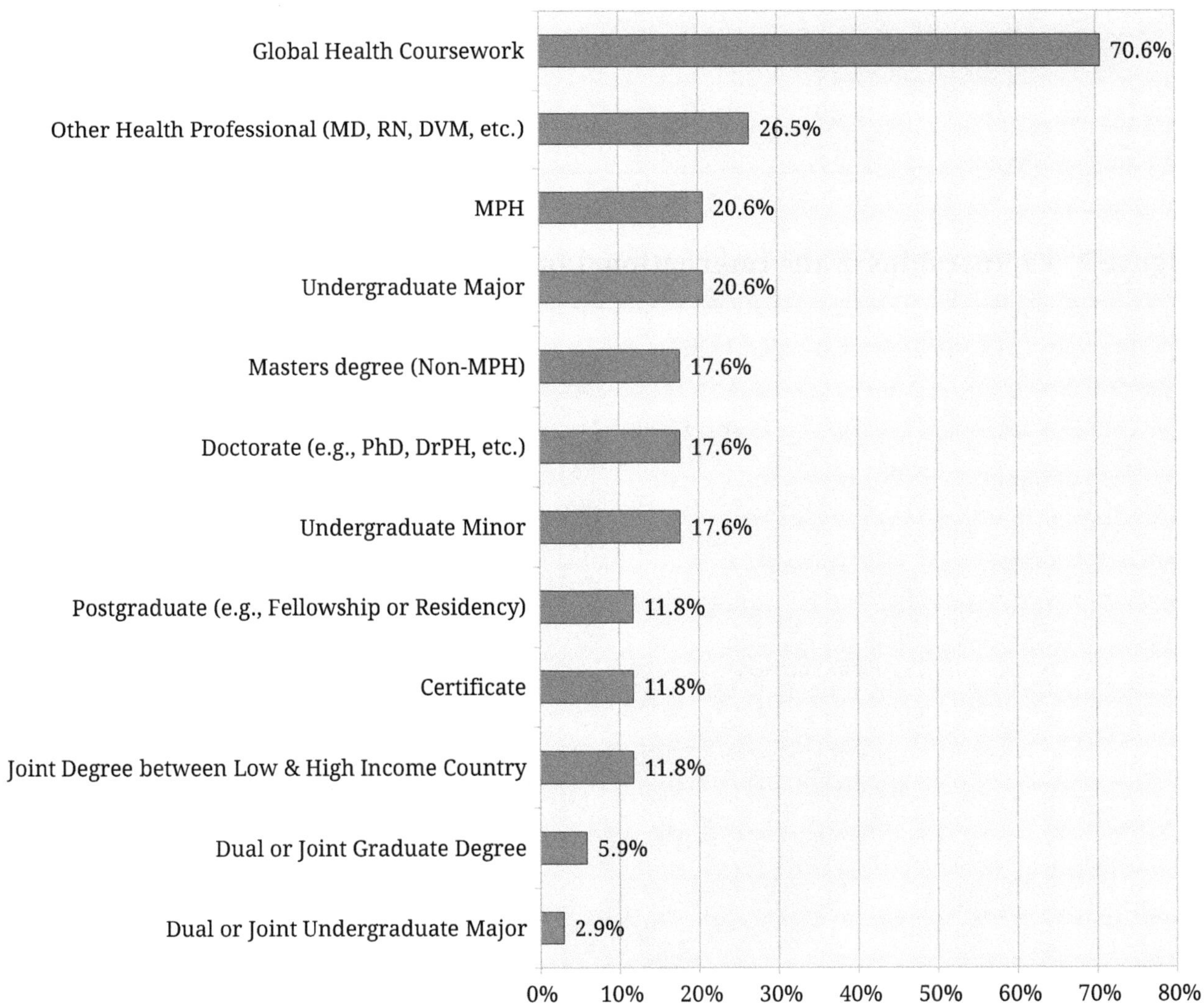

Finally, Figure 8 shows the degree of importance of funding sources that international partner institutions reported as being particularly critical for the success of their global health partnerships with North American academic institutions.

The most important funding sources (listed as Essential or of High Importance) were the North American universities themselves, followed by international research agencies (such as NIH and IDRC). Although PEPFAR and MEPI funding was not received by more than half of the international partners surveyed, these were separately identified as Essential or High Importance funding sources by about 40 percent and 30 percent, respectively, of those surveyed. Funding from other North American government agencies such as USAID and CIDA, UN agencies, and international NGOs and foundations were rated as either essential or highly important by roughly 40 percent of those surveyed.

Table 3. Number of Partnerships per International Partner Institution, n = 37

	n (%)
1	5 (13.5)
2–5	8 (21.6)
6–10	11 (29.7)
11–15	5 (13.5)
16–20	5 (13.5)
20+	3 (8.1)

Figure 7. Partnerships of the International Institutions by Region, n = 516

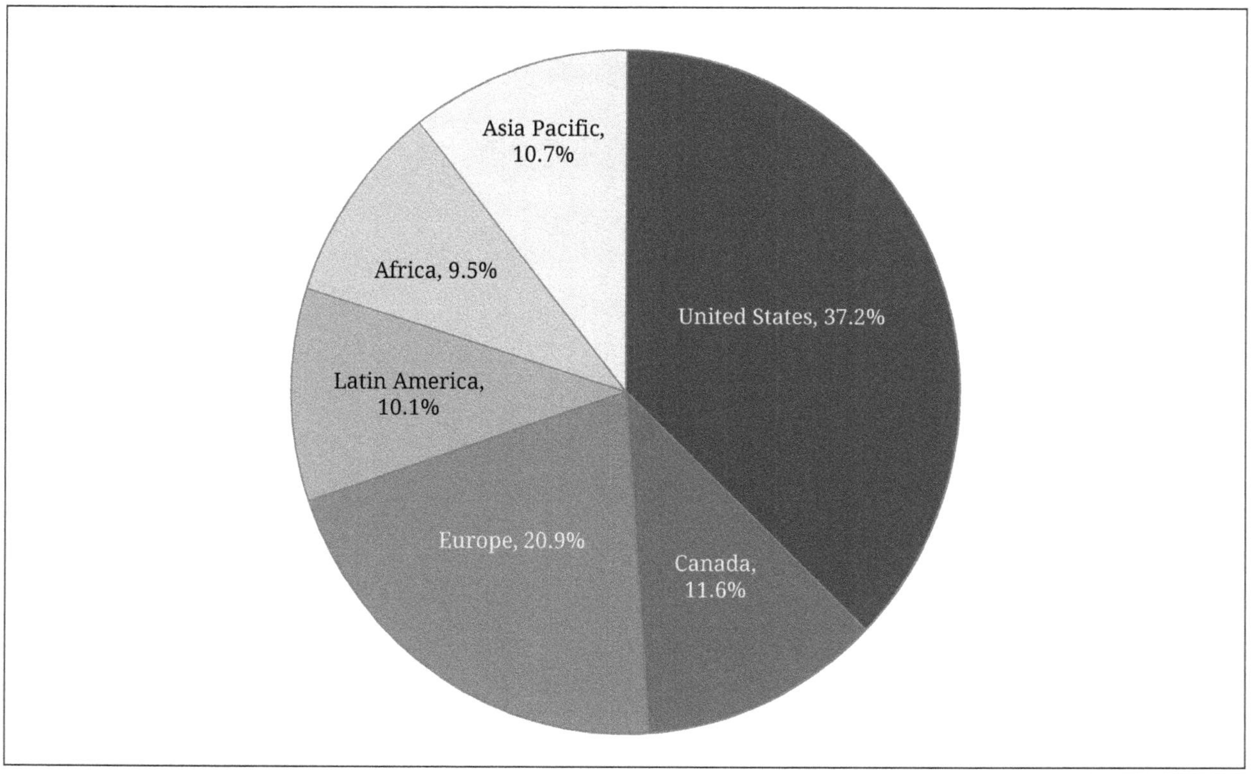

Figure 8. Importance of Funding Sources for International Partner Institutions (International Partner Survey), n = 38

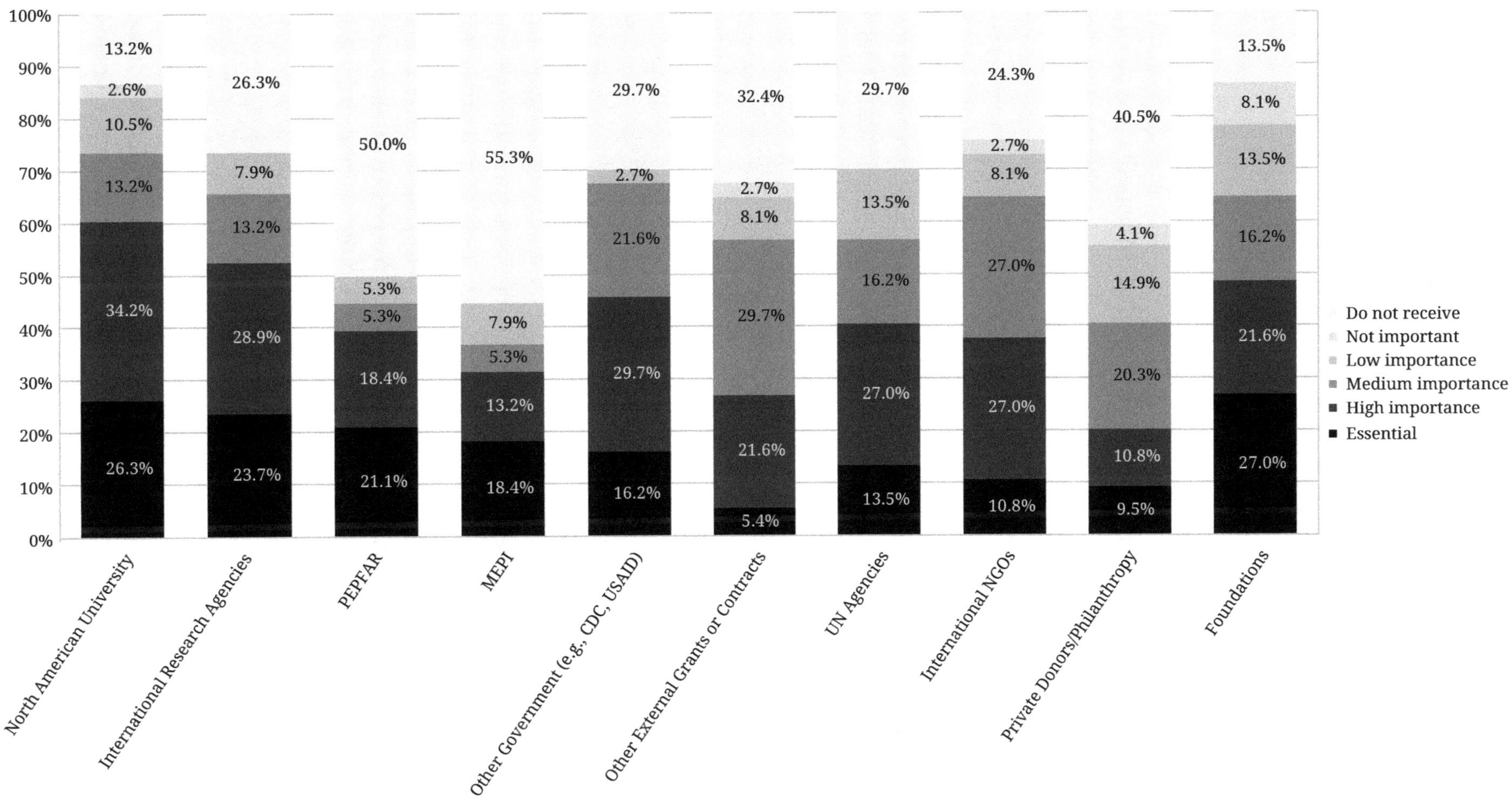

1 | Assessing Global Health Partnerships

Evaluating the mutual benefits and the determinants of benefits, harm, equity, and sustainability of global health partnerships generated a variety of findings within and between groupings of North American and international partner institutions.

BENEFIT AND HARM

Three activities were selected for detailed analysis: *Research Collaboration, Education and Training*, and *Global or Local Health Impact. Research Collaboration* and *Education and Training* were selected for more detailed presentation due to their high level of focus as reported by all respondents in this study as well as in the earlier CSIS/UW report on university global health programs.[1] Given that positive health impact is arguably the ultimate goal of global health programs, Global Health Impact is also included.

Research Collaboration

Collaboration on research is the most frequently reported collaboration among global health partners as reported both by North American academic institution and by international partner respondents (Figure 3 and Figure 9). Over 90 percent of North American academic institution respondents reported engaging in research collaboration with their international partner institutions, and 79.5 percent of international institutions reported engaging in research collaborations with North American academic institution partners (Figure 9).

Research collaborations are also widely perceived as being highly beneficial to all partnership members. The majority (over 80 percent) of North American academic institution respondents reported that research collaborations are either *Very Beneficial* or *Beneficial* to their programs. Over 80 percent of North American academic institution respondents also reported that they perceive that research collaborations are either *Very Beneficial* or *Beneficial* for their partners (Figure 10). This perception is likewise held by the international institution respondents, with over 75 percent reporting research collaborations as either *Very Beneficial* or *Beneficial* for their own institution. Such consistency across survey respondents suggests a relatively high level of equity in benefits derived from research collaborations among the majority of global health partnerships represented by our data.

1. Matheson et al., "Sustainability and Growth of University Global Health Programs."

Figure 9. Types of Partnerships with North American Academic Institutions (International Partner Survey), n = 39

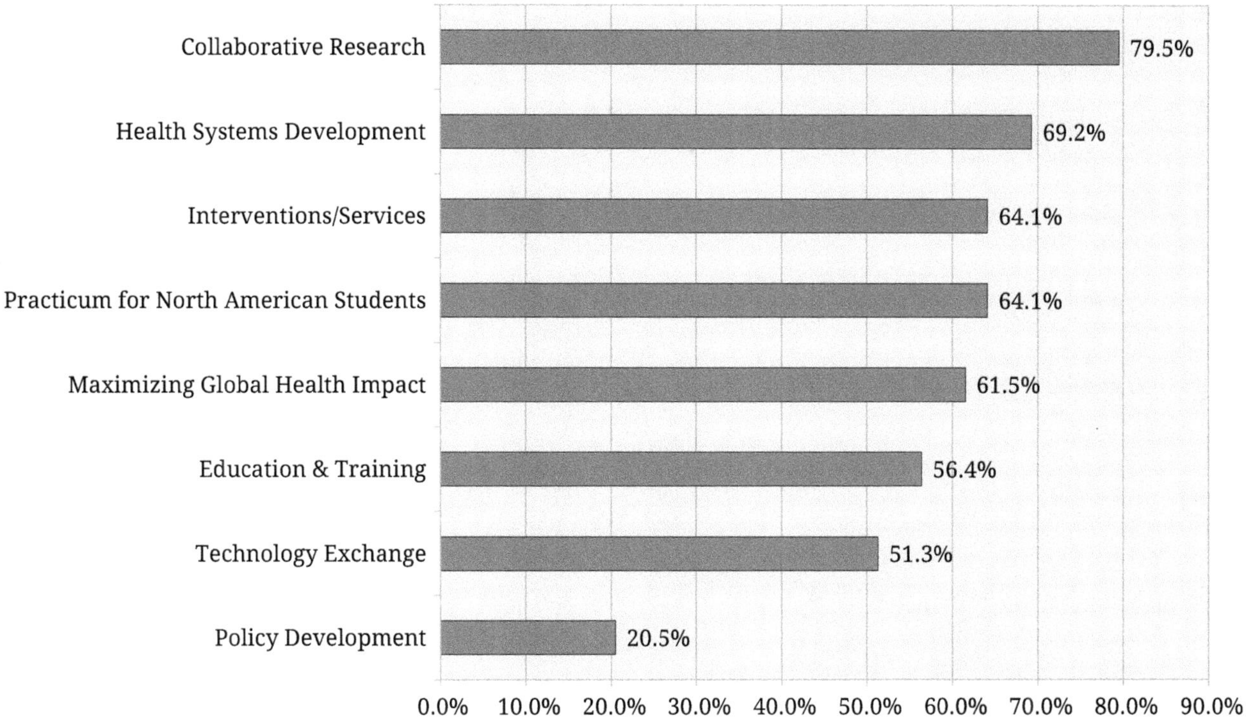

The importance and benefit of research collaboration was woven throughout interview responses as well, both from North American and from international respondents. Many of the international respondents described their ability to leverage their international research collaborations to gain independent funding. Interview respondents also expressed the benefit from increased opportunities to tap international experts in other countries for research support and collaboration as well as for networking and professional development opportunities. Moreover, one international institution professor explained that research collaboration and the ensuing publications had helped his institution to "identify ourselves somewhere in the global map."

Education and Training

Education and training, particularly for the next generation of global health experts, was cited as a substantial focus of academic global health programs in the *Sustainability and Growth of University Global Health Programs* report.[2] It was also frequently emphasized in the published case studies reviewed. A similar pattern reflecting this focus on education and training was observed throughout this study. Of the top four categories of partnership activities reported by North American academic institutions, three relate to education, training, or learning experiences (see Figure 3), with each of these education-related categories reported by about 80 to 90 percent of North American academic institution respondents.

2. Ibid.

Figure 10. Perceptions of Global Health Partnership Benefits from Research Collaborations

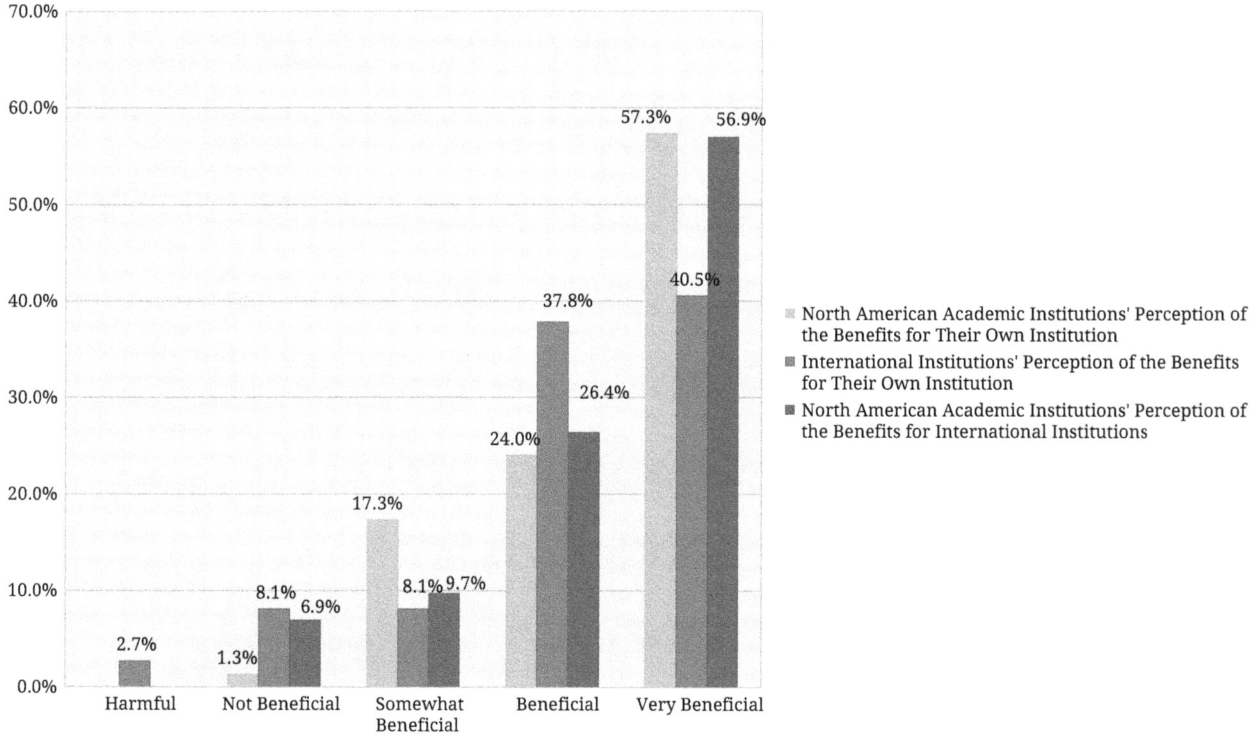

Given the focus on education, it is perhaps not surprising that nearly 90 percent of North American academic institutions reported global health partnerships as either *Very Beneficial* or *Beneficial* to student knowledge acquisition within their academic programs (see Figure 11). Similarly, roughly 80 percent of North American academic institutions reported that they perceive that their global health partnerships are either *Very Beneficial* or *Beneficial* for their international partners in areas of knowledge acquisition, training, and mentoring. Among interview respondents, all were able to name a number of educational benefits to their own institutions stemming from international partnerships. Most North American respondents cited opportunities for their students to engage in educational experiences outside of North America as one of the greatest benefits of international partnerships, both through gaining a greater understanding of health problems and service delivery in low-resource settings and as a professional development opportunity. A number of respondents also described the importance of on-site mentors to make student trainee exchanges a logistic and educational success. Collaborative nonclinical health systems training is also taking place; one North American global health leader described an upcoming bidirectional program with a West African country partner in which faculty from both sides will be trained in monitoring and evaluation.

International institutions reciprocated these perceptions. The majority (81 percent) reported international partnerships as either *Very Beneficial* or *Beneficial* for their own students' knowledge acquisition (see Figure 11) and also for their faculty knowledge acquisition (89.1 percent, data not shown), despite the overall paucity of mechanisms to send their

Figure 11. Perceptions of Global Health Partnership Benefits in Regards to Student Knowledge Acquisition

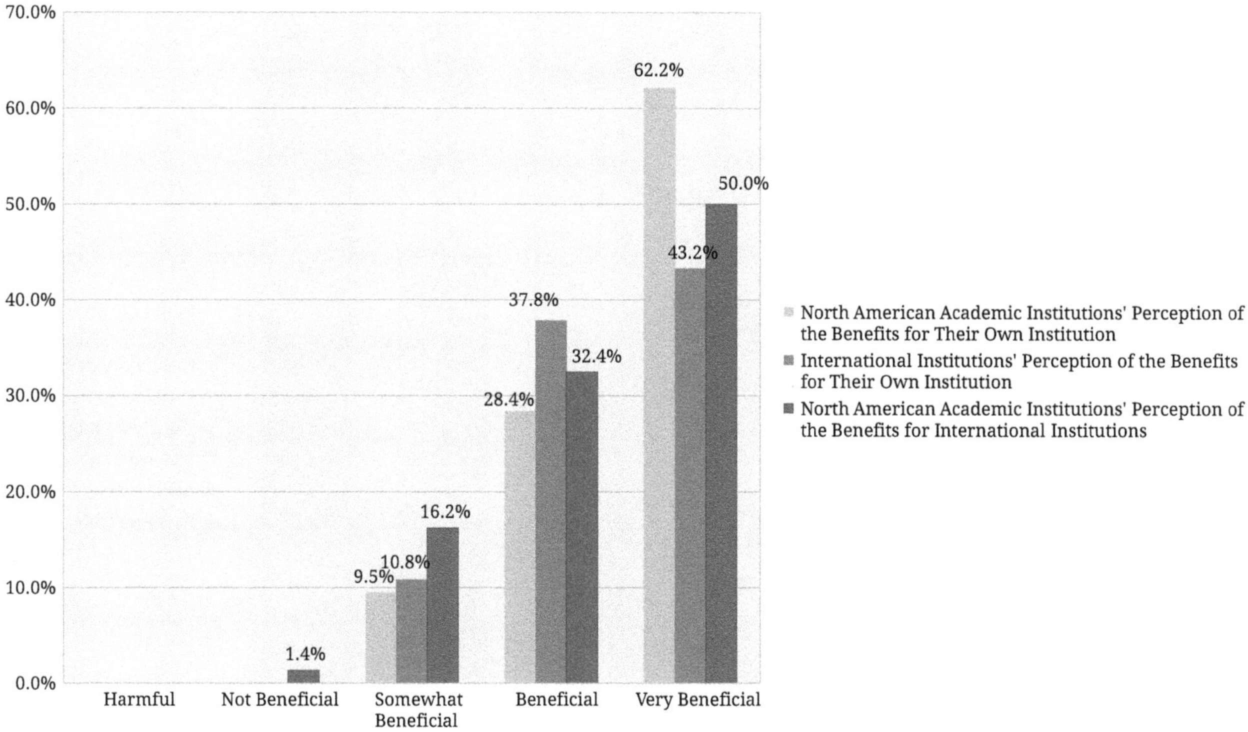

own students and faculty to North America for exchanges. In interviews, international respondents often cited the benefit of interacting with North American faculty members to learn more about teaching strategies and curriculum development. International mentorship between faculty members in global health partnerships was highly valued, and multiple international respondents described how these types of relationships with North American researchers could further the careers of young researchers in low-income settings. As one researcher in East Africa explained: “Collaboration has created experts through mentorship . . . [and] through mentorship these experts are able to create systems.” Another echoed this response: “Somebody young goes to another university and comes back to create a bridge.” Both North American and international respondents emphasized that faculty knowledge acquisition is bidirectional and that North American faculty do benefit and learn new skills that they can take back to their home institutions. Further benefits may be derived from the knowledge that North American students acquire; when international interview respondents were asked what they saw to be the benefits of partnerships to North American academic institutions, the majority responded that they saw exposure of North American students to the health problems not endemic in North America, such as malaria and tuberculosis, as the main or sole benefit. Additionally, some international respondents described the benefits to their own students of working with North American partners in the international respondents’ home country through connections made and exposure to Western culture, should they travel abroad after their studies. This has implications for future partnerships and greater global health impact.

Figure 12. Evaluation of North American Student Training, by Category of Training (North American Academic Institution Survey), n = 75

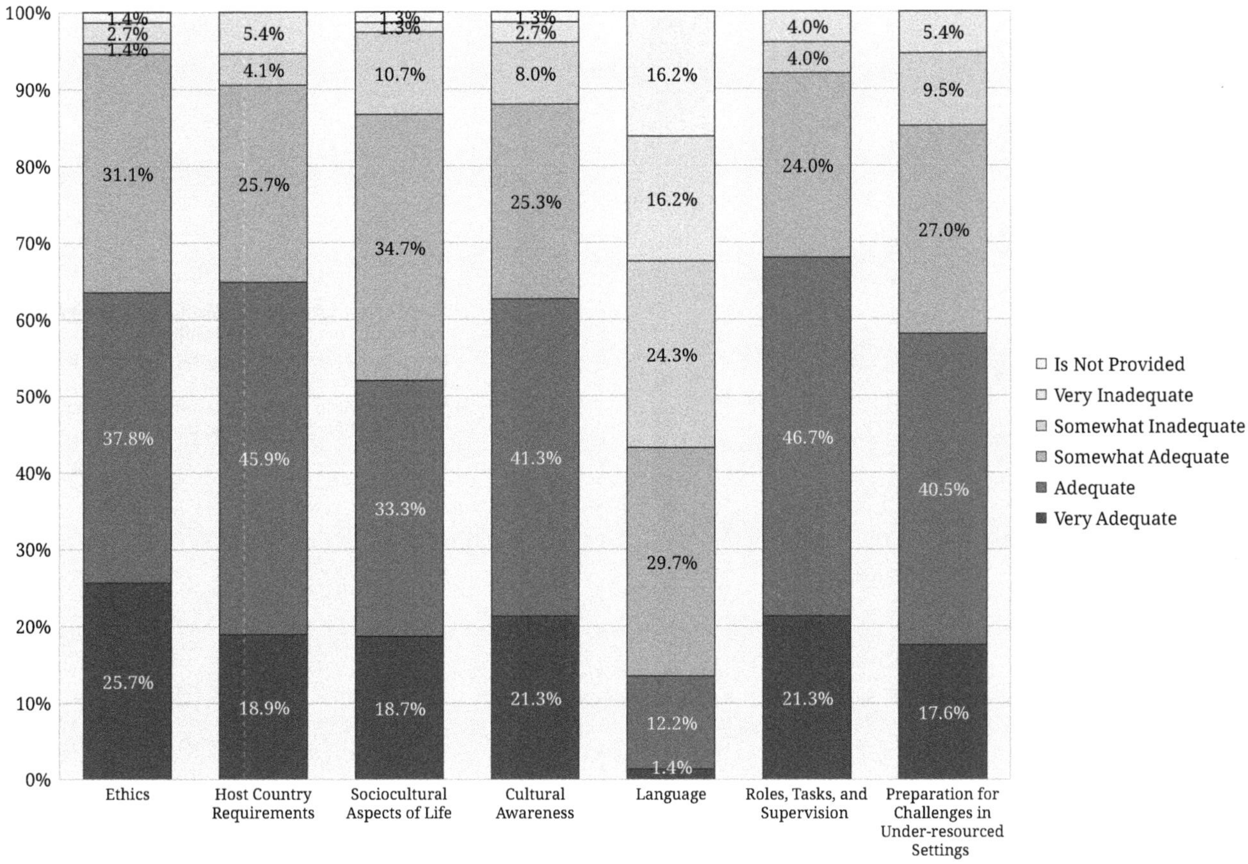

Although both North American academic institutions and international institution partners reported educational and training outcomes as beneficial to their programs, perceptions regarding the adequacy of student training and preparation were more varied. While roughly 80 percent of all North American academic institution respondents (Figure 12) and of international institution respondents (Figure 13) rated the education and training of North American students as *Somewhat Adequate*, *Adequate*, or *Very Adequate* in almost all categories, both groups acknowledged that language training remains an area of concern. Moreover, while North American academic institution respondents thought the cultural awareness of their own students was satisfactory (more than 60 percent considered this *Adequate* or better), global partners were less satisfied (only 41.7 percent of international respondents considered North American students *Adequate* or better in cultural awareness, and 41.7 percent rated this awareness as only *Somewhat Adequate*). In offering suggestions for how North American students can better prepare for experiences abroad, most international partners indicated that even limited amounts of culture and language training could go a long way. Common suggestions including placing more emphasis on providing background on the culture and customs of the settings of students' destinations before arriving, bolstering language training when feasible, and increasing awareness of visiting students of the challenges and limitations of working in low-resource settings. As one respondent succinctly put it, "They shouldn't expect North America in Africa."

Figure 13. Evaluation of North American Student Training Preparation, by Category of Training (International Institutions Survey), n = 36

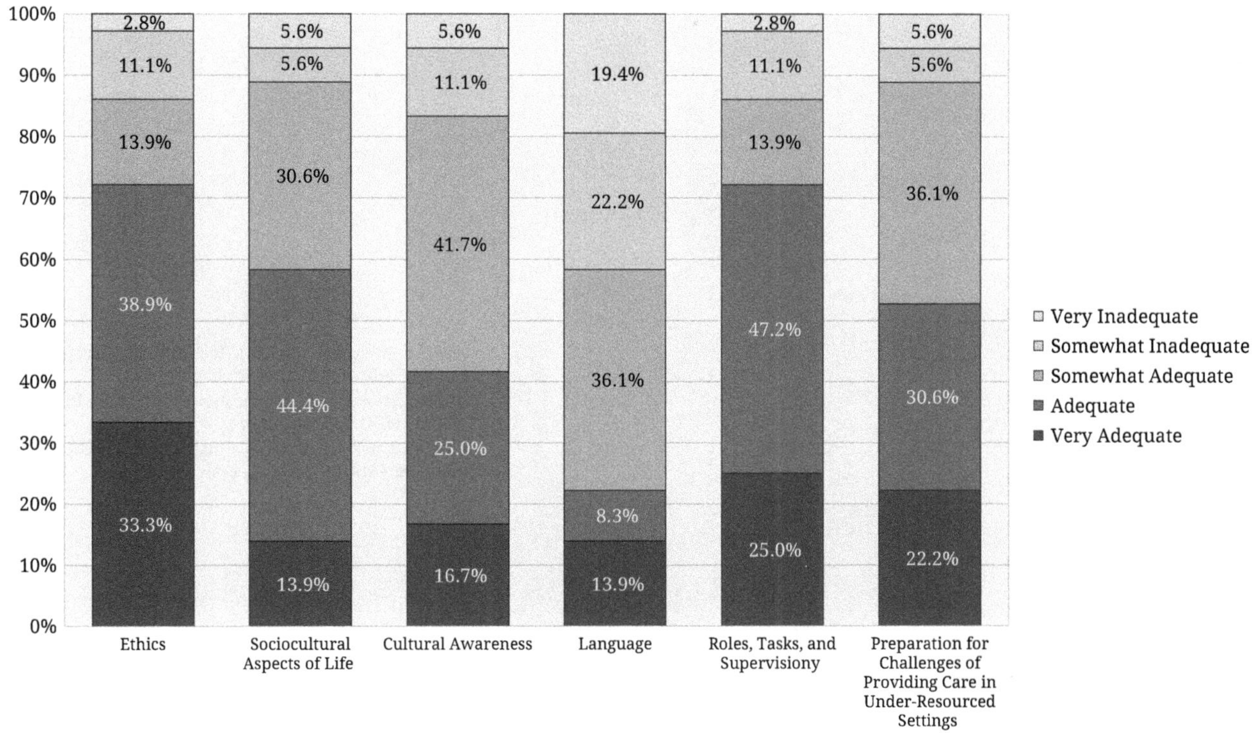

Global Health Impact

The majority of North American Academic Institution survey respondents (75 percent) reported that global health partnerships are either *Very Beneficial* or *Beneficial* to maximizing their own programs' global health impact (Figure 14). Sixty percent of North American institutions thought that global health partnerships are either *Very Beneficial* or *Beneficial* for global health impact for their partners; similarly, just under 60 percent of international partners reported that global health partnerships are either *Very Beneficial* or *Beneficial* to their own global health impact. However, global health impact was perceived as *Very Beneficial* almost twice as often by North American academic institutions (40 percent) than by international institution partners (18.9 percent).

Overall, both the North American and international partners rated the research and education benefits of their collaborations higher than the health impact benefits. For instance, 40 percent of North American academic institution respondents reported their own program's global health impact was *Very Beneficial*, whereas 62.2 percent reported student knowledge acquisition was *Very Beneficial*, and 57.3 percent reported research collaboration was *Very Beneficial*. Similar trends are noted for international partners. The lower ratings for global health impact may partly reflect the fact that global health partnerships are relatively young and the time from creating a new program or intervention until achieving impact may be quite long.[3] However, it may be that some partnerships do not

3. Health Economics Research Group, Office of Health Economics, RAND Europe, *Medical Research: What's it worth? Estimating the economic benefits from medical research in the U.K.* (London: U.K. Evaluation Forum, 2008).

Figure 14. Perceptions of Global Health Partnership Benefits in Regards to Health Impact

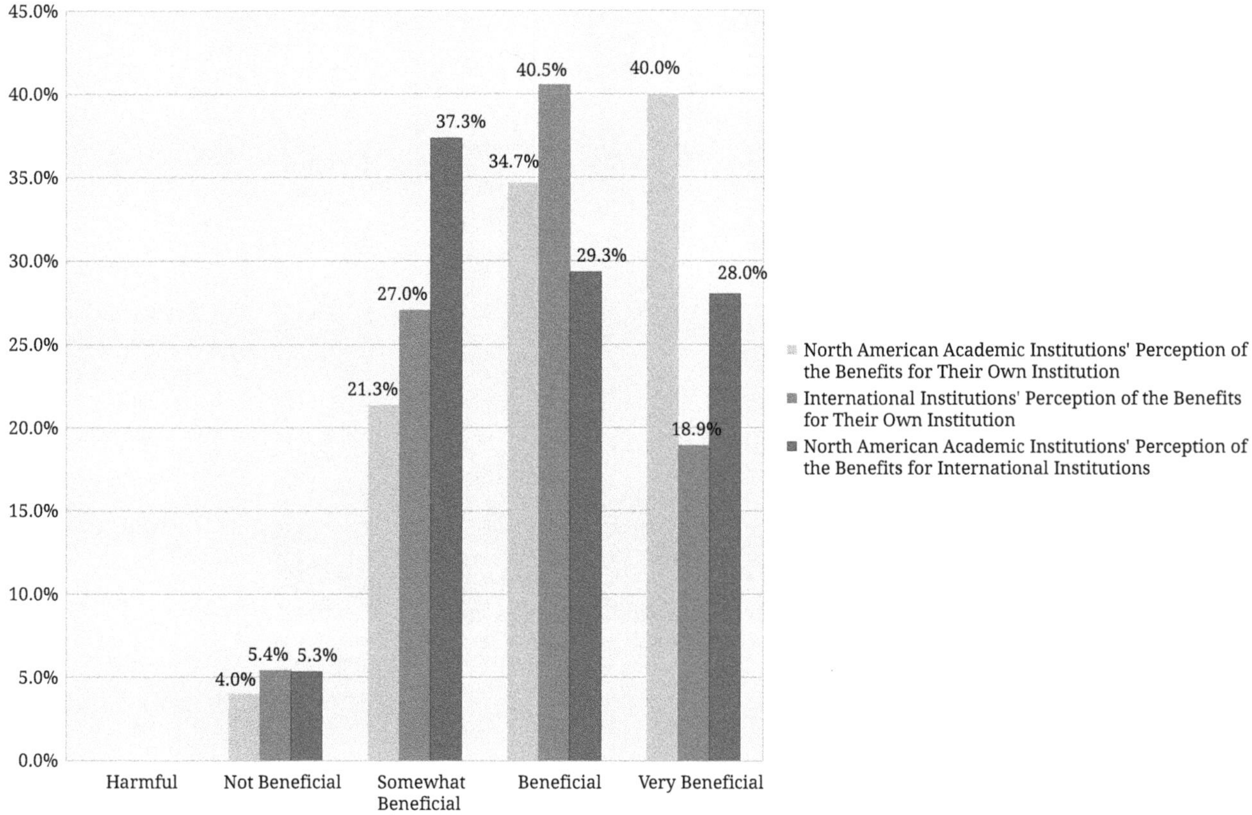

ultimately achieve high health impact. One global health leader expressed that she was "not sure yet about impact. We have to evolve. There is a need of creating global health leaders, and they can't just be from the [global] North, but must also be from the [global] South." As a caveat, it is important to note that strong mechanisms for systematically measuring health impact over time are not yet fully developed or universally employed. Future reassessments over time may show clearer evidence of whether or not there is higher global health impact across all three categories: research, education, and health impact.

Global Health Justice and Equity

Global health programs and their impact should address reducing health disparities and improving health equity and justice for all communities. In interviews, respondents were asked how they conceptualized global health justice and equity, and if or how it was reflected in the impact of their work and their partnerships. All respondents agreed on the importance of these goals and overwhelmingly discussed both justice and equity in terms of reducing health disparities. One North American global health leader defined it as follows: "The goal of justice and equity is to ensure that the benefits of society are accessible to everybody, at every level." Another respondent asserted that while their institution did not "brand" itself around justice and equity per se, both are so inherently intertwined with global health as to be a given in global health programs. Some respondents cited specific focus areas where they felt that justice and equity were particularly realized in their work: for example, in advancing human rights, reducing HIV stigma, and conducting clinical trials for drugs to treat neglected tropical diseases. How a continuing focus on global health justice and equity can best influence further global health impact remains an important goal of global health partnerships.

Harm

It is encouraging to report that global health partnerships were rarely reported as being perceived as harmful—*fewer than 3 percent of North American academic institutions or international institutions reported any type of partnership activity as "harmful."* However, it remains important to examine the mutual responsibilities required in partnerships, as well as the overall effectiveness of foreign aid as an intervention in low- and middle-income countries. Within the wider global health context, concern has been expressed that global health work can create harm through creating dependence (and therefore hampering sustainability), distorting host country salaries, and putting a burden on facilities and care providers to provide support for North American trainees when resources are already stretched thin.[4] Out of 82 surveys from North American academic institutions in which potential harm was explicitly addressed by the survey, only one respondent (1.3 percent) reported a perception that partnerships focusing on health systems strengthening might be harmful for their international partners, and another reported that global health partnerships might be harmful with respect to funding diversification (data not shown), but no other aspect of any of the other partnerships was perceived to be harmful. With respect to surveys of the international partners, of 34 survey respondents, only one (2.9 percent) reported that any aspect of their partnership was harmful (with respect to research support as seen in Figure 8, as well as with respect to financial support, intervention services, technology exchanges, and student exchanges; data not shown). *While harm was minimally reported in the surveys and not mentioned in interviews, we cannot fail to mention the need to prospectively address potential risks that may come with international global health programs.*

Apart from explicit harm, somewhat more common were perceptions that partnership activities were only somewhat beneficial or not beneficial at all, suggesting that even when harm is not an issue there is still room for improvement. For example, research collaborations were reported as only *Somewhat Beneficial* or *Not Beneficial* by 18.6 percent of North American academic institutions and 16.2 percent of international institutions, while the same was reported for education and training by 9.5 percent of North American institutions and 10.8 percent of international institutions. In addition, 25.3 percent of North American institution and 32.4 percent of international institution respondents reported that global health partnerships are only *Somewhat Beneficial* or *Not Beneficial* to maximizing their programs' global health impact.

---

4. T. L. Hall et al., "Global Health 'Actors' and Their Programs," Consortium of Universities for Global Health (presented at the UCSF Global Health Education Consortium, San Francisco, April 14, 2011).

FACTORS CORRELATED WITH PERCEIVED BENEFITS

In interviews with leaders at both North American academic and partnering international institutions, several factors (e.g., funding and institutional support) were reported as associated with more beneficial partnerships. These factors were assessed for their broader relevance using survey data (see Tables 4 and 5 for descriptive statistics of all survey data used in this study) in univariate regression analyses (see Tables 6 and 7 for analyses results). Three dependent variables were used in assessing factors associated with increased benefits: the NAAI Self Benefits Scale, the NAAI Benefits to Partners Scale, and the IPI Self Benefits Scale (this report's Methods section provides a detailed description of all variables included in the statistical analyses).

Of all the factors identified as important in global health partnerships, funding was the most frequently discussed and was often depicted as crucial to success—"more funding equals more possibilities." Conversely, multiple global health leaders also stated that "[lack of] funding is always a barrier." These assertions were corroborated by statistical analyses in which the importance of various forms of funding were positively associated with perceptions of increases in partnership benefits for both North American academic and international institution respondents.

Beyond funding, multiple respondents discussed the need for institutional support. "You need to have university support at all levels; without support [partnerships are] not going to be successful." The importance of institutional support was supported by statistical evidence; for example, for North American academic institution programs, being part of larger university partnerships (interpreted as having access to larger institutional collaboration and support) was positively and significantly associated with greater reported benefit.

Student training in preparation for gaining global health experience was also mentioned by several global health leaders as important to partnership success; as one respondent explained, "Students are your best resource, but you also can't ask them to do things that they are not trained to do." Similarly, international partner respondents noted that students were not always well prepared for the challenges of working in resource-limited locations and that this can detract from partnership success. Statistical analyses support these assertions; perceptions of the adequacy of North American student training were positively associated ($p = 0.001$) with increases in international institutions reporting benefit to their own institution.

Global health leaders at North American academic institutions and at international institutions also agreed that strong interpersonal relationships and communication, as building blocks to effective and efficient collaborations, are vital to deriving partnership benefits. Statistical analyses support these assertions; that is, the factor *Collaboration Assessment* was positively associated with increases in reported benefit by both North American academic and international institutions, although only statistically significant for the North American academic institutions.

Table 4. Descriptive Statistics for Survey Data from North American Academic Institutions (NAAI)

Dependent Variables	Min	Max	Mean Value	Percent
NAAI Self Benefits Scale	20	35	29.1	—
NAAI Benefits to Partners Scale	18	40	31.7	—
NAAI Collaborations Scale	12	36	25.2	—
Independent Variables	Min	Max	Mean Value	Percent
NAAI Funding Value				
University Funding	1	6	2.4	—
NIH Funding	1	6	3.1	—
PEPFAR Funding	1	6	4.3	—
Other Government Funding	1	6	3.3	—
External Grants/Contracts	1	6	3.4	—
Private Donor Funding	1	6	3.3	—
Foundation Funding	1	6	3.2	—
NAAI Funding Scale	7	42	27.5	—
NAAI NIH Funding Amount				
<10 million	—	—	—	17.9
10 million–49.9 million	—	—	—	26.9
50 million–200 million	—	—	—	34.6
>200 million	—	—	—	20.5
NAAI Endowment				
<100 million	—	—	—	9.2
100 million–999.9 million	—	—	—	28.9
1 billion–5 billion	—	—	—	40.8
>5 billion	—	—	—	21.1
NAAI Private	—	—	—	41.5
NAAI Part of Larger Institutional Partnerships	—	—	—	68.5
NAAI Enrollment				
<2,500	—	—	—	9.0
2,500–9,999	—	—	—	12.8
10,000–40,000	—	—	—	59.0
>40,000	—	—	—	19.2
NAAI Scope of Coursework, Certificate, Major, or Degree Offerings	1	12	4.6	—
NAAI Assessment of North American Student Training Scale	8	36	26.5	—
NAAI Collaborations Scale	12	36	25.2	—

Note: Scale variables were recoded from lowest to highest ratings. For example: **NAAI Self Benefits** combines the ratings of perceived benefits in seven areas, each area recoded as 1 = Harmful, 2 = Not Beneficial, 3 = Somewhat Beneficial, 4 = Beneficial, 5 = Very Beneficial; **NAAI Benefits to Partners** combines the ratings of perceived benefits in eight areas, each area recoded as 1 = Harmful, 2 = Not Beneficial, 3 = Somewhat Beneficial, 4 = Beneficial, 5 = Very Beneficial; **NAAI Collaborations** combines the ratings of how well a program is working together with its international partners in six areas, recoded as 1 = Not Done, 2 = Poor, 3 = Fair, 4 = Well, 5 = Very Well, 6 = Excellent; **NAAI Funding** includes seven different funding sources, each recoded as 1 = Do Not Receive, 2 = Not Important, 3 = Low Importance, 4 = Medium Importance, 5 = High Importance, 6 = Essential; **NAAI Funding** combines the ratings of the seven different funding sources.

Table 5. Descriptive Statistics for Survey Data from International Partner Institutions (IPI)

Dependent Variables	Min	Max	Mean Value	Percent
IPI Self Benefits Scale	22	45	34.2	—
IPI Collaborations Scale	7	30	20.1	—
IPI Needs Fulfillment	7	39	23.9	—
Independent Variables	Min	Max	Mean Value	Percent
IPI Funding Source				
North American University	1	6	2.7	—
NIH	1	6	3.1	—
PEPFAR	1	6	3.9	—
MEPI Funding	1	6	4.2	—
Other Government	1	6	3.3	—
External Grants/Contracts	1	6	3.8	—
UN Agencies	1	6	3.5	—
NGO	1	6	3.4	—
Private Donor	1	6	4.0	—
Foundation	1	6	3.0	—
IPI Funding Scale	11	60	37.4	—
IPI—Collaborations and Investments Received	0	6	2.7	—
IPI—Type of Institutions				
Private Academic	—	—	—	61.7
NGO	—	—	—	10.6
Government Agency	—	—	—	19.2
Other Agency	—	—	—	8.6
IPI Scope of Coursework, Certificate, Major, or Degree Offerings	0	7	1.8	—
IPI Assessment of North American Student Training Scale	6	26	19.3	—
IPI Collaborations Scale	7	30	20.1	—

Note: Scale variables were recoded from lowest to highest ratings. For example: **IPI Self Benefits** combines the ratings of perceived benefits in nine areas, each area recoded as 1 = Harmful, 2 = Not Beneficial, 3 = Somewhat Beneficial, 4 = Beneficial, 5 = Very Beneficial; **IPI Collaborations** combines the ratings of how well a program is working together with its North American partners in five areas, each area is recoded as 1 = Not Done, 2 = Poor, 3 = Fair, 4 = Well, 5 = Very Well, 6 = Excellent; **IPI Needs Fulfillment** combines the ratings of how well global health partnerships are fulfilling the institutional needs of international institutions in seven areas, each area is recoded as 1 = Not Done, 2 = Poor, 3 = Fair, 4 = Well, 5 = Very Well, 6 = Excellent; **IPI Funding** includes 10 different funding sources, each recoded as 1 = Do Not Receive, 2 = Not Important, 3 = Low Importance, 4 = Medium Importance, 5 = High Importance, 6 = Essential; **IPI Funding** combines the ratings of the 10 different funding sources.

EQUITY

Equity was a strong and recurring theme in both survey and interview responses. In the surveys, multiple indicators were used in assessing the overall equity of global health partnerships, and these were complemented by interview questions that targeted similar topics. We explore the emergent themes in three sections below: collaboration, benefits to international partners, and comparing perceptions of benefit.

Table 6. Factors Associated with North American Academic Institutions' Perceptions of Benefits from Global Health Partnerships for Their Institutions and Partnering International Institutions

	NAAI Self Benefits Scale		*NAAI Benefits to Partners Scale*	
Independent Variable	*Relationship*	*p-value*	*Relationship*	*p-value*
NAAI Funding Source	+	**<0.001**	+	**<0.001**
University Funding	+	0.3	+	**0.01**
NIH Funding	+	**0.008**	+	**<0.001**
PEPFAR Funding	+	**0.007**	+	0.07
Other Government Funding	+	**0.03**	+	**0.008**
External Grants/Contracts	+	**0.01**	+	**0.005**
Private Donor Funding	+	0.2	+	0.2
Foundation Funding	+	**0.001**	+	**<0.001**
NAAI NIH Funding Amount	+	**0.05**	+	**0.05**
NAAI Endowment	+	0.2	+	0.1
NAAI Private	+	0.08	+	**0.007**
NAAI Part of Larger Institutional Partnerships	+	**0.01**	+	**0.003**
NAAI Enrollment	–	0.8	–	0.5
NAAI Scope of Coursework, Certificate, Major, or Degree Offerings	–	0.5	–	0.2
NAAI Assessment of North American Student Training	+	0.4	–	0.9
NAAI Collaborations Scale	+	**<0.001**	+	**0.001**

Note: Additional information for each variable is outlined in the Methods section.

Collaboration

North American academic institutions and international institutions were asked to assess how well they are collaborating with their global health partners in five areas:

- Assessing the Needs of International Institutions
- Establishing Mutual Goals
- Addressing the Needs of International Institutions
- Planning, Monitoring, and Evaluating the Impact of Collaborations
- Soliciting or Providing Feedback

Despite our own initial concerns about potential inequities, and concerns expressed by a global health colleague[5] that some global health partnerships reflect characteristics of "neocolonialism," our surveys and interviews actually found that most North American

5. This colleague was not directly involved in this study.

Table 7. Factors Associated with International Institutions' Perceptions of Benefits from Global Health Partnerships for their Institutions

	IPI Self Benefits Scale	
Independent Variables	*Relationship*	*p-value*
IPI Funding Source	+	**0.003**
North American University	+	**0.002**
NIH	+	**0.03**
PEPFAR	+	0.3
MEPI Funding	+	0.2
Other Government	+	0.2
External Grants/Contracts	+	0.08
UN Agencies	+	**0.05**
NGO	+	0.07
Private Donor	+	0.08
Foundation	+	**<0.001**
IPI—Collaborations and Investments Received	+	**<0.001**
IPI—Type of Institutions*		
Private Academic	–	0.9
NGO	+	0.9
Government Agency	+	0.4
Other Agency	+	0.4
IPI Scope of Coursework, Certificate, Major, or Degree Offerings	+	0.5
IPI Assessment of North American Student Training	+	**0.001**
IPI Collaborations Scale	+	**0.02**

Note: Additional information for each variable is outlined in the Methods section.
*Public academic institutions are reference category.

academic institutions and international partner institutions were collaborating well with their partners. Over 60 percent of North American academic institutions and international partners rated their partnership collaborations as working *Well, Very Well*, or *Excellent* for each of the five areas. It is noteworthy that international partners were more likely than North American academic institutions to rate their collaboration as *Excellent* for all areas, except for addressing the needs of international partners. These findings speak to the importance of collaboration and communication in establishing mutual goals, monitoring and evaluating impact, or evaluating progress through feedback—all of which was echoed in interviews.

Setting specific goals early in the process of collaboration was the "best practice" most frequently voiced by interview participants. In particular, it was mentioned by the majority of international participants, both as a way to set expectations and a means of "[avoiding] situations where you are taking things as you can get them." Indeed, a shared vision that encompasses the needs of both partners and speaks to both short- and long-terms goals is seen as the underpinning of a successful collaboration. In assessing how well they are working with their international global health partners in establishing mutual goals, over

Figure 15. Evaluation of How Well Global Health Partners Are Working Together in Establishing Mutual Goals

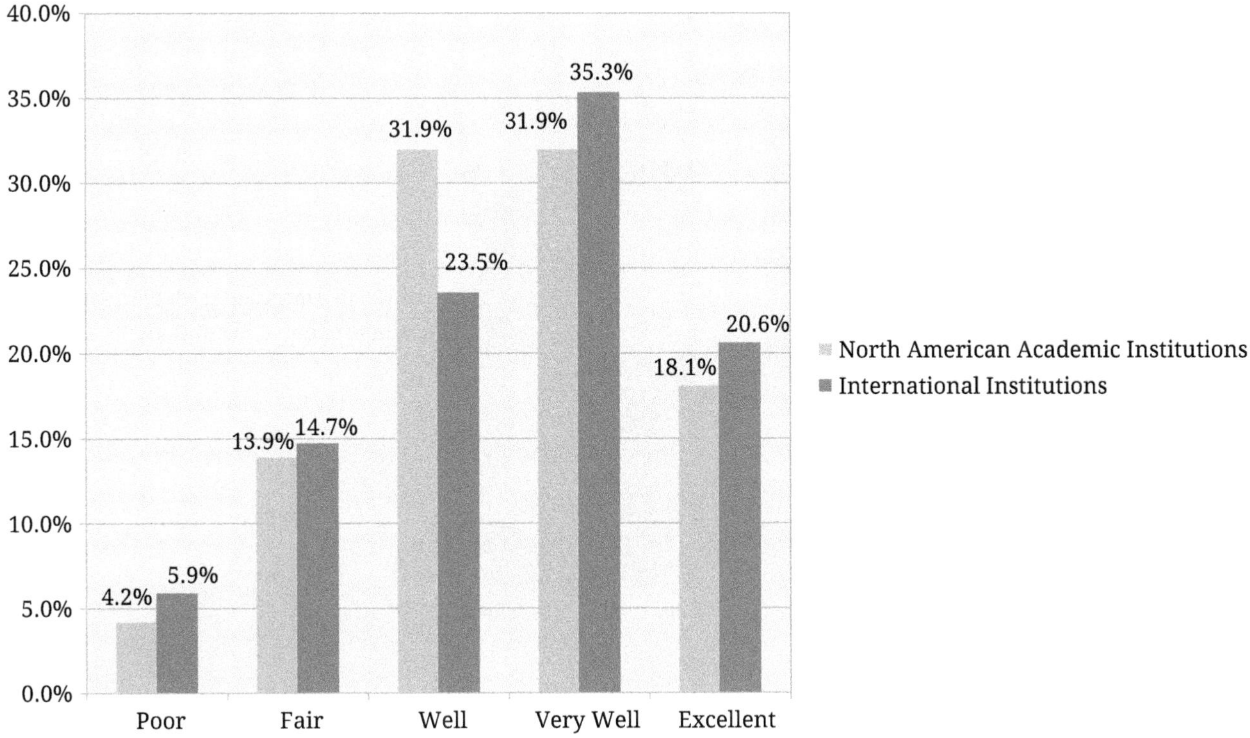

three-quarters of North American academic institutions and international institutions respondents reported their collaborations as working *Well*, *Very Well*, or *Excellent* (see Figure 15); conversely, only 3 percent to 4 percent reported their collaborations as working poorly. This pattern is consistent with the high level of importance that interviewees ascribed to establishing mutual goals in their partnerships and indicates that both North American academic institutions and international institutions recognize the importance of establishing mutual goals and are actively working together to make this a reality.

However, in going beyond establishing mutual goals, it is important to monitor and evaluate the impact of collaborations in achieving these goals.[6] The surveys suggest that this has been more difficult to accomplish (Figure 16). Monitoring and evaluation mechanisms ranged from nonexistent to informal to formal, and were an issue or concern noted most frequently by North American respondents. Many specifically cited their lack of a formal evaluation system and/or the need for improvement in this area. These respondents explained that evaluation occurs informally or as needed, but that a more systematic approach would be valuable. However, a number of North American respondents did give examples of more formal evaluation methods. One described a system in which students and on-site mentors complete evaluations after each exchange. In addition, students communicate directly with on-site partners for letters of support and to establish scopes of work in order to increase the partners' investment and mutual understanding. Another

6. M. L. Rosenberg et al., *Real Collaborations: What It Takes for Global Health to Succeed* (Oakland: University of California Press, 2010).

Figure 16. Evaluation of How Well Global Health Partners Are Working Together in Monitoring and Evaluating Impact

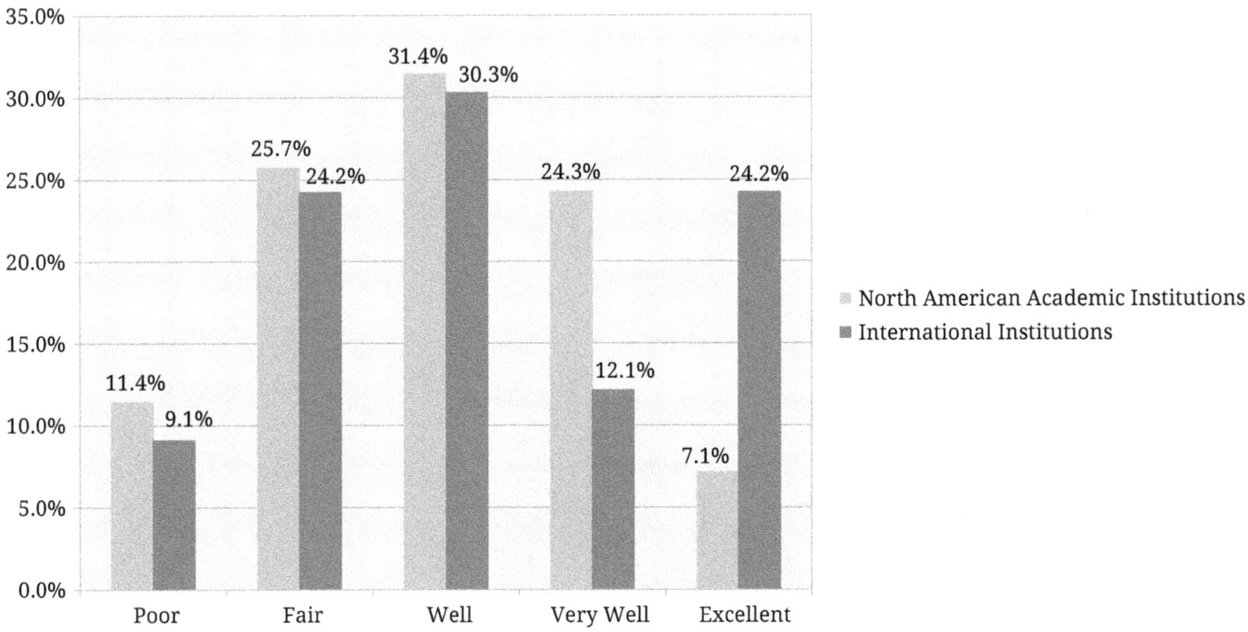

program described an online management system that is used within the university and with partners to facilitate assessment and evaluation while also providing a platform for the development and exchange of teaching and curriculum materials. Finally, one institution described a regular evaluation and ranking process that prioritizes international partnerships based on the following criteria: externally funded research; whether medical residents and other graduate and undergraduate students are regularly engaging with the international partner institution by traveling to the partner's location; whether multiple disciplines are involved; and whether a memorandum of understanding is in place.

The broader surveys were consistent with the interviews, indicating that efforts among partners to monitor and evaluate impact vary substantially. While over 60 percent of North American academic institution and international institution respondents reported that they were working *Well* or better with their global health partners in monitoring and evaluating impact (Figure 16), the percentage of international institutions that reported that their working relationship with North American partner institution was *Excellent* was higher than vice versa (24.2 percent compared to 7.1 percent). Conversely, North American academic institution respondents reported slightly more often than international institutions that efforts in working together on monitoring and evaluation were either *Fair* or *Poor*. These survey findings are consistent with reports from interviewees who noted that the practice of monitoring and evaluation ranges from nonexistent to informal to formal. In seeking to improve monitoring and evaluation efforts, many respondents recognized the importance of efficient and effective communication between global health partners.

Communication through e-mail, Skype, cell phones, and other means has made regular contact feasible. Few respondents in North American academic institutions or

Figure 17. Evaluations of the Perceptions of North American and International Institutions on How Well They Are Working Together as Global Health Partners in Soliciting or Providing Feedback

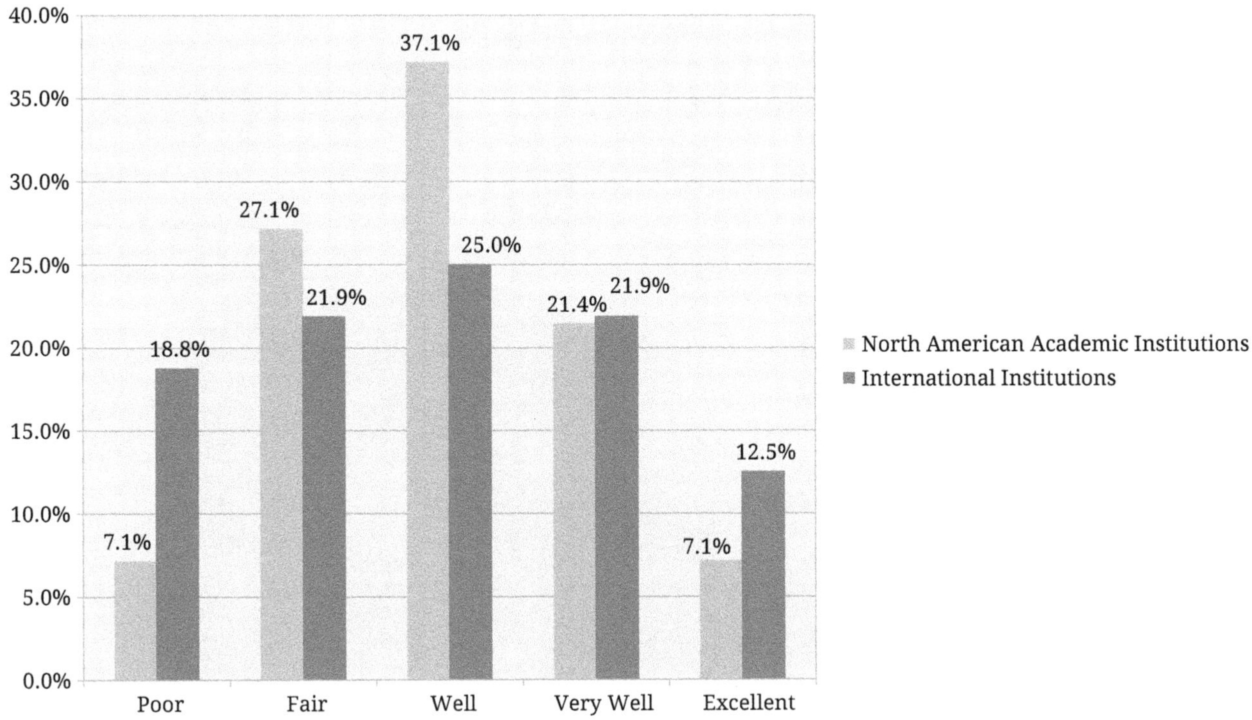

international institutions mentioned difficulty in reaching partners. Still, many explained that even frequent e-mail communication cannot replace the importance of more personal methods of communication, whether through phone calls or especially site visits with face-to-face interaction. One international respondent described the benefits of biweekly conference calls with his institution's North American partner: "Even though we are so far apart, we each know exactly how things are happening at any given time." Both North American and international respondents cited personal relationships as important underpinnings of good communication. One professor at an international university explained, "We are human beings, we are social creatures, so it is easier for us when we have this type of interaction." Another international partner echoed this view: "Personal relationships that you build during training are the key aspect . . . once you have that you can start building." On the North American side, in-person interaction was valued as well. As one North American professor noted, "You can't conduct international research from a desk."

As one measure of communication, survey respondents were asked to evaluate how well they were either soliciting feedback or providing feedback to their partners (see Figure 17). The near-perfect bell curve distribution of responses show a wide range in partnership communication for both North American academic institution and international institution respondents, indicating considerable room for improvement by systemizing communication.

Figure 18. Ratings by International Partners of Fulfillment of their own Institutional Needs, n = 32

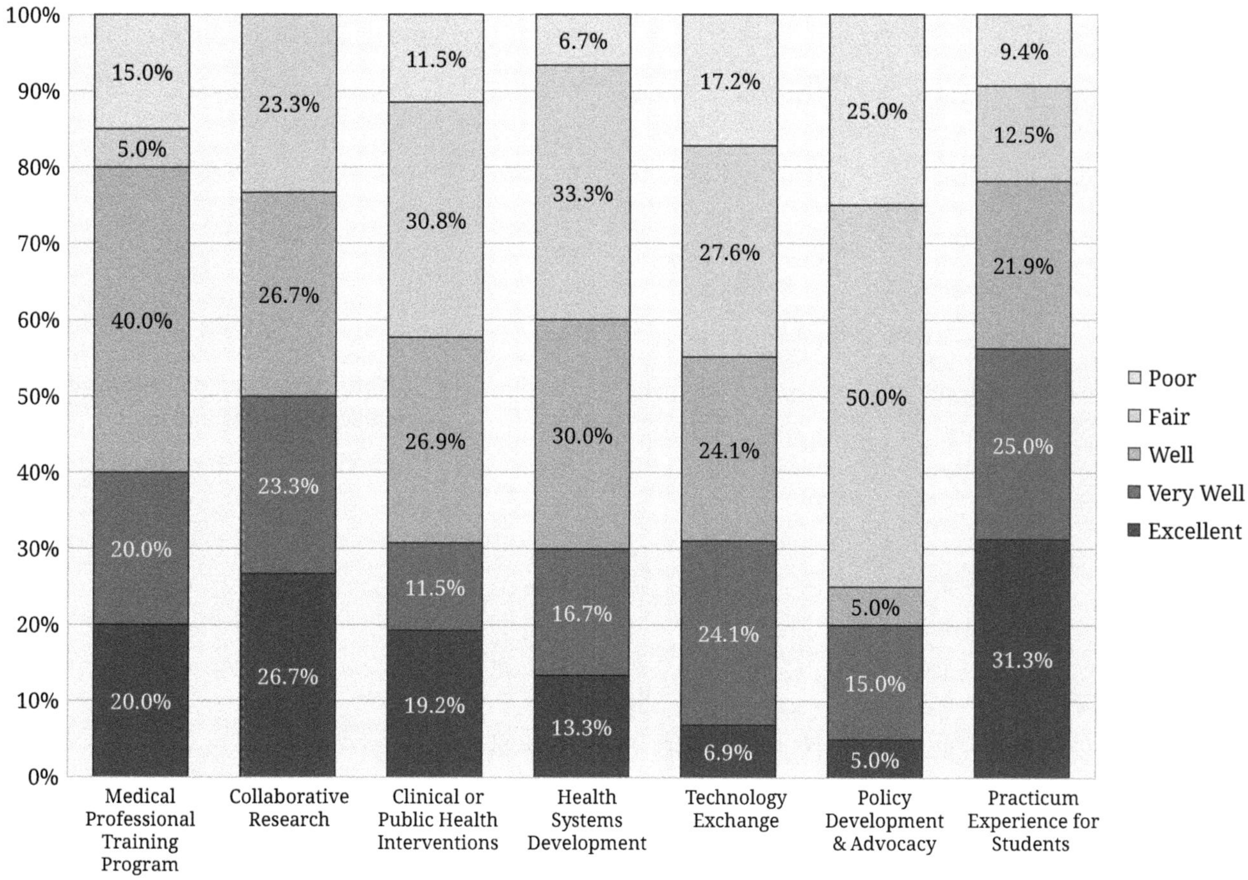

Benefits to International Institutions

Evaluating the extent to which international institutions reported that their specific institutional needs were being fulfilled gives additional insight into where global health partnerships are likely succeeding in providing equitable benefit to international partners (see Figure 18).

An assessment of the ratings by international institutions of how well their partnerships fulfilled their own institutional needs (Figure 18) shows a pattern that echoes the findings for partnership benefits. Over 70 percent of respondents representing international institutions reported that their institutional needs were being fulfilled at the *Well*, *Very Well*, or *Excellent* level for needs related to either Research Collaboration or Education (i.e., Research Collaborations, Medical Professional Training Programs, and Learning and Practicum Experiences for Students). In interviews, global health leaders at international institutions described grant-writing support, assistance with curriculum development, and development of collaborative research projects as key benefits from their partnerships.

However, these collaborations were perceived as less successful with respect to health impact and policy development and advocacy. For needs closely aligned with realizing

Figure 19. International Partners' Assessment of the Adequacy and Usefulness of Collaborative Investments from North American Partners, n = 38

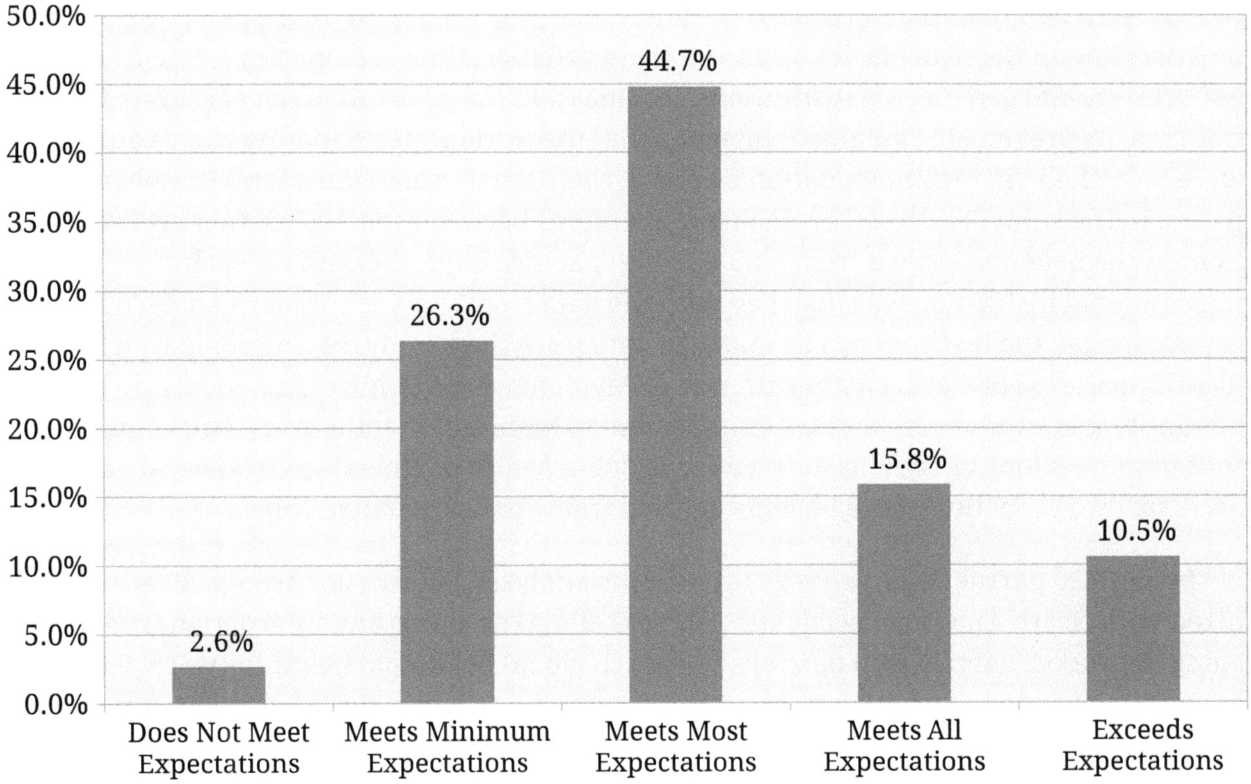

local health impact in international settings (i.e., Clinical or Public Health Interventions, Health Systems Development, Technology Exchange, and especially Policy Development and Advocacy), fewer international respondents rated fulfillment for these activities at the highest level (*Excellent*) compared to their ratings for educational or research outcomes. The ratings of benefits for technology exchange were also surprisingly modest. The least beneficial area is seen for Policy Development and Advocacy, where only 25 percent of survey respondents rated their needs as favorably fulfilled. This was echoed in interview findings. This may be an area for potential improvement, even though local leadership is particularly important in Policy Development and Advocacy.

Despite differences in fulfillment of needs across these indicators, the majority (71 percent) of international partners reported that the collaborative investments (e.g., student training, cash resources, collaborative research grants, support for curriculum development) they received from their North American partners met *Most* or *All Expectations*, or even *Exceeded Expectations* in terms of adequacy and usefulness (see Figure 19). While this is encouraging, 26.3 percent of international partners reported that collaborative investment only met *Minimum Expectations*, and 2.6 percent stated it *Does Not Meet Expectations* at all.

COMPARING PERCEPTIONS OF BENEFIT

In aggregate, both North American academic and international institutions were generally favorable in their assessment of how well they were working with their global health partners and in the benefits derived from these collaborations. Comparing perceptions between specific partnering institutions provides additional detail to the aggregated findings. As previously explained, international institutions participating in this study were identified via recommendation by one of their North American partners also participating in the study. To directly compare perceptions between specific partnering institutions of the benefits derived from global health partnerships, the data for each international institution was matched with the data from the North American partner that recommended the institution. The matched data were then analyzed and compared to identify patterns of similarity or difference. Partners were not identified, to ensure confidentiality and candid responses. It is important to highlight that these are still comparisons of perceptions of benefits derived from global health partnerships in general and not necessarily a reflection of the benefits derived from specific partnerships.

In total, 30 partnership pairings inform this analysis. Figures 20 through 26 are organized with North American academic partners along the x-axis and international partners along the y-axis. Partnership pairings for which global health partnerships were perceived as equally beneficial by both partners are represented as white circles, partnership pairings for which the North American partner perceived greater benefits than were perceived by their international partner are represented as dark gray circles, and partnership pairings for which the international partner perceived greater benefits than were perceived by their North American partner are represented as light gray circles. Circle size represents the number of partnership pairings at a specific rating.

These figures give further evidence that, in general, global health partnerships are perceived as beneficial for all categories of benefit examined both by North American academic and by international institutions; that is, between 50 percent to 100 percent of all of the partnership pairings are in the range of *Somewhat Beneficial*, *Beneficial*, or *Very Beneficial*. However, they also indicate that when perceptions among partnering institutions do differ, North American academic institutions more often rate global health partnerships as more beneficial for their international partners (Figures 20 to 24) and for their own institutions (Figures 25 and 26) compared to rankings by the international partners of their own benefits.

This is exemplified with respect to the perceived benefits that international institutions derive from research collaborations with North American partners (Figure 20). Within 31 partnership pairings, 12 partnerships (white) reported identical perceptions of benefit resulting from research collaborations. However, North American academic institutions rated perceived benefits to the international partner higher than the perceived benefit ratings by the international partner in 13 instances (dark gray); but conversely, the international partners rated their perceived benefits higher than did the North American partners in only 6 instances (light gray). Overall, 70 percent of partnership pairings were rated by

Figure 20. Comparison of Benefits for International Partners from Research Collaborations as Perceived by the International Partners Themselves and as Perceived by Their North America Partners

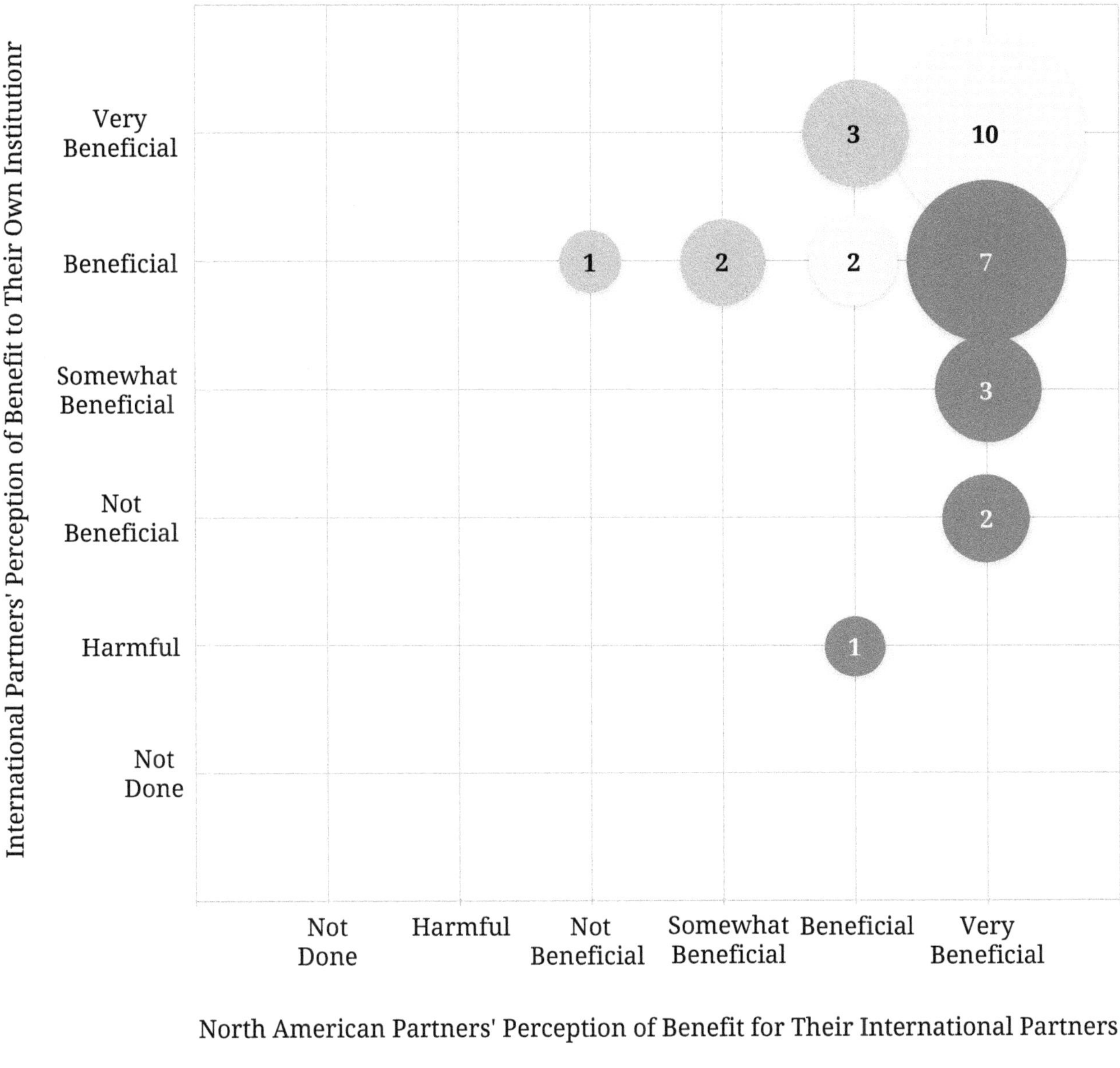

both partners as either *Very Beneficial* or *Beneficial* for the international partners. Similar distributions are seen in Figures 21 to 23.

In contrast to the other comparisons, perceptions of the benefits that international institutions derive from student exchanges are more varied (Figure 24), with more rankings for either *Not Beneficial* or *Harmful*. This finding, while unfortunate, is in line with perceptions reported in interviews with global health leaders at both North American academic and international institutions in which there was a general perception that student exchanges often are less beneficial for international institutions, with fewer students traveling to North American institutions than vice versa.

Figure 21. Comparison of Benefits for International Partners from Student Knowledge Acquisition as Perceived by the International Institutions Themselves and as Perceived by Their North America Partners

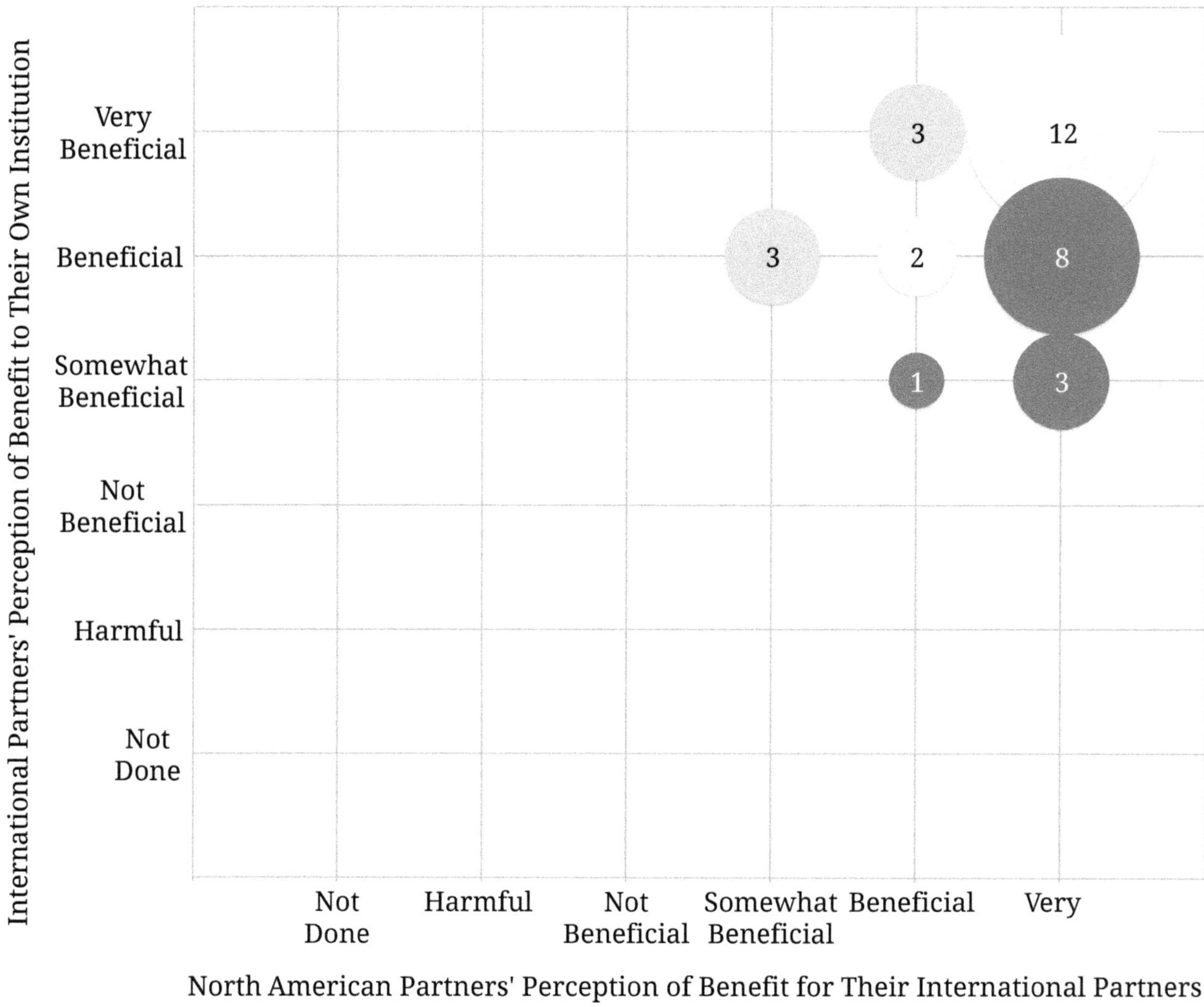

In addition, Figures 25 and 26 indicate that for some categories of benefit, North American academic partners somewhat more often perceived greater benefit than was perceived by their international partners. For student knowledge acquisition (Figure 25), the North American and international partners gave the same rating (*Beneficial* or *Highly Beneficial*) in 13 instances; the North Americans gave higher ratings in 13 instances, and international institutions gave higher ratings in 6 instances. A similar distribution was seen in ratings of benefits in global health impact (Figure 26).

Multiple North American respondents acknowledged that some level of inequality is inevitable in partnerships with institutions in lower-resource settings. Much of this stems from funding and financing, which most commonly flows from the global North to South and from resources such as technologies, which were greater in North American institutions. While the flow of funding and technologies from North to South can potentially benefit the South, a principle concern with disparities in funding and other resources is

Figure 22. Comparison of Perceived Benefits for International Partners in Terms of Global Health Impact as Perceived by the International Partners Themselves and as Perceived by Their North American Partners

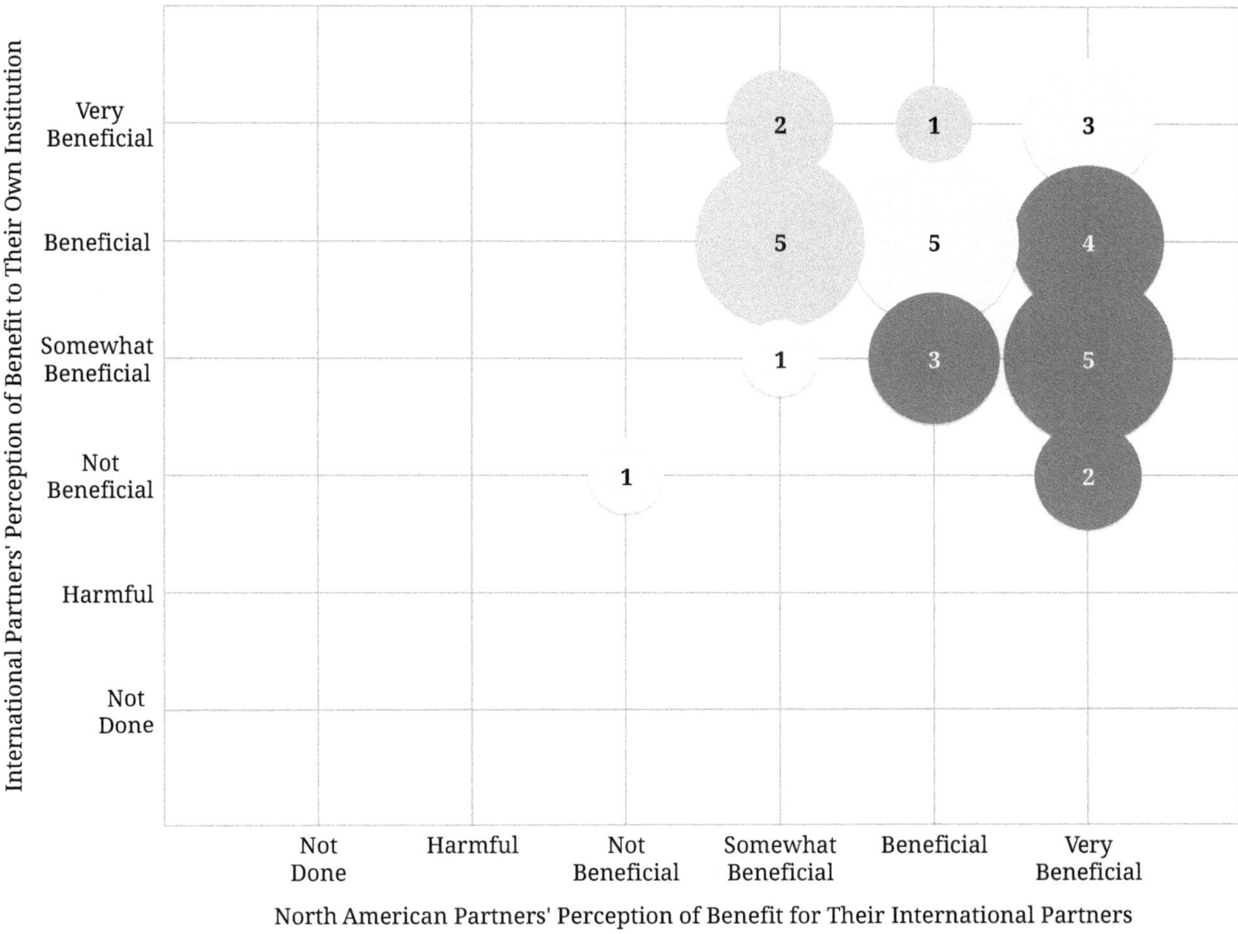

that they lead to unequal power in decisionmaking between the partners. In interviews with global health leaders, differences in perception of benefits were manifested primarily in the lack of bidirectionality in student exchange. Many student exchanges within partnerships are not bidirectional, and it is often much easier for U.S. students to go abroad for various reasons (especially financial and access to visas). Among international partners interviewed, very few were currently sending their students to U.S. institutions for short- or long-term study or had concrete plans to do so. The difficulty of achieving true bidirectional exchange within partnerships means that, as one dean at a university with a large U.S. global health program said, "sometimes that feeling of true reciprocity is challenged." As another dean explained, "The fact of the matter is sometimes it is an uneven playing field . . . [and] if you don't keep your eye on the ball it can start to feel very unequal." She described U.S. students traveling to foreign countries with travel grants provided by their home institution and staying for no cost at their host institution's medical campus. There is no housing equivalent at this respondent's U.S. institution, and most foreign students do not have access to travel grants. A second respondent echoed the observation that it is very easy for North American students to travel abroad, but much more

Figure 23. Comparison of Benefits for International Partners from Financial Support as Perceived by the International Partners Themselves and as Perceived by Their North American Partners

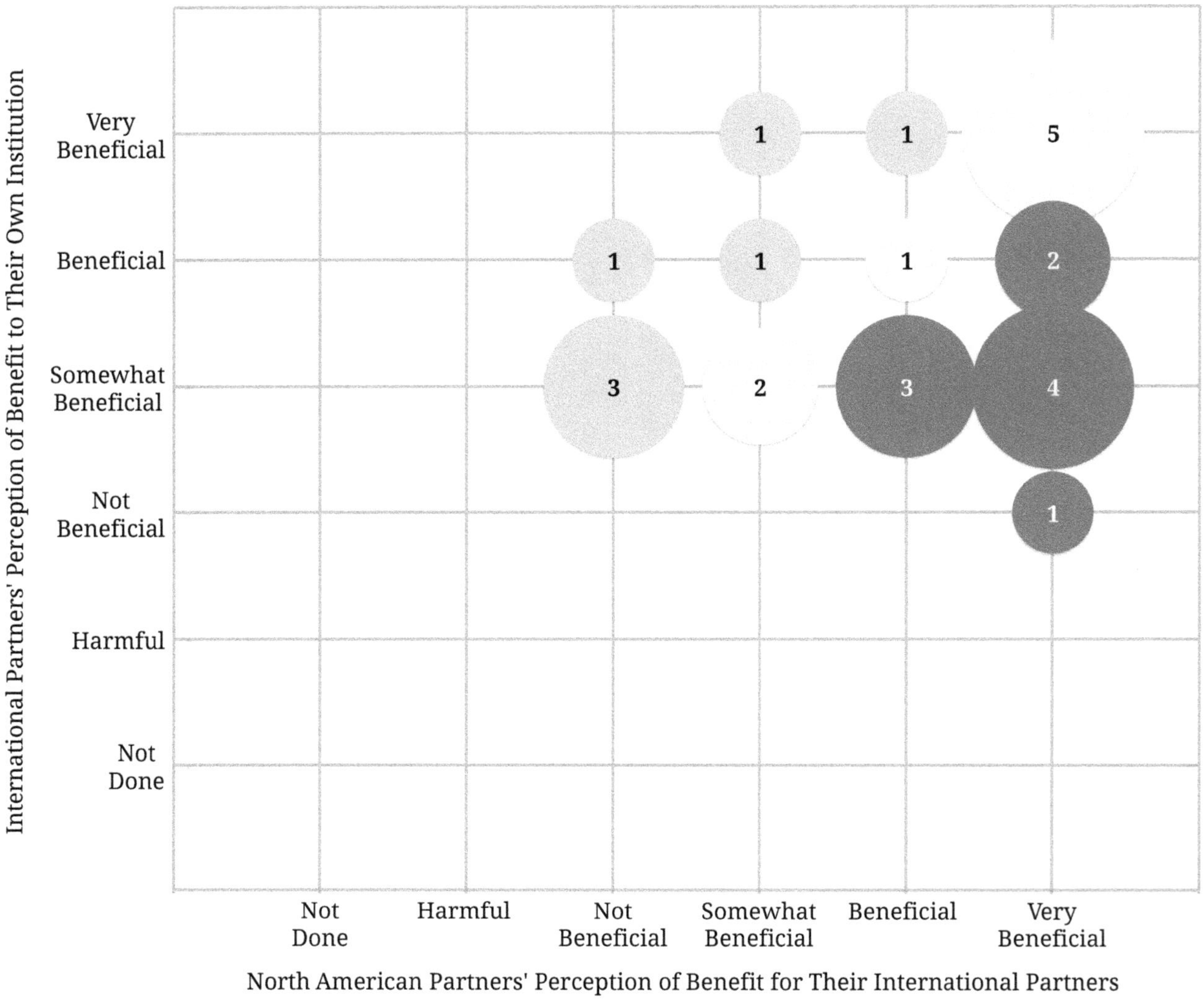

difficult for students from low- and middle-income countries to travel to North America to study. A third respondent, a professor at a university in North Africa, described the difficulty of exchanges: "To take students to the U.S., it is almost impossible. Even for a visa, our students are expected to pay six or seven times the visa cost of what a North American student pays to come to our country." He added that it is often much easier for students from his university to undertake exchanges or rotations with European partners because of more favorable regulations. Funding is just one of many barriers to bidirectional exchange; the policies of the academic institution, state laws that prevent clinical work by international trainees, training grants that may be restricted to U.S. citizens, and English language requirements are all factors that make it difficult for international students to study in North America.

Beyond financial imbalance and concerns about student exchanges, there was a perception among international interview respondents that partnerships are not always equal,

Figure 24. Comparison of Benefits for International Partners from Student Exchanges as Perceived by the International Partners Themselves and as Perceived by Their North American Partners

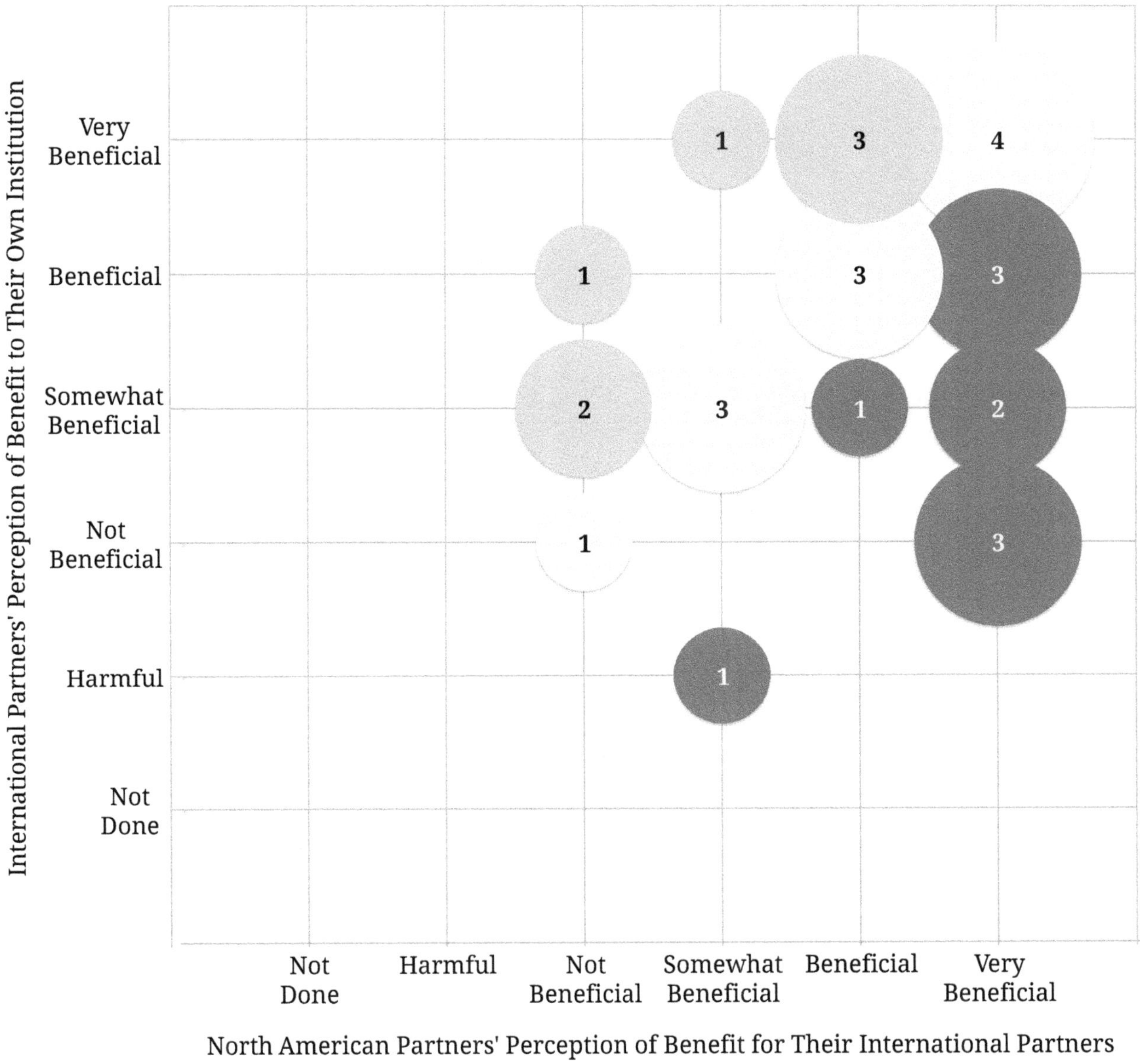

and some don't address equity. One respondent described the frustration of grant money being eaten up in administrative costs before it left their North American partner institution, stating, "We are not getting as much as we should." Another described a situation in which his organization collects data but their North American partner analyzes it, therefore preventing his organization from building analysis and laboratory capacity. As he described, "Because we do not have technical capacity, we are limited by how much we can do with the samples that we collect . . . research in [the respondent's country] is generally problem-driven whereas in the U.S. it is university-driven." Two international respondents described a recurring problem of North American researchers coming to their country, conducting research, and then not including host-country collaborators in research publications.

Figure 25. Comparison of Benefits to Their Own Institution from Student Knowledge Acquisition as Perceived by North American Academic Institutions and as Perceived by Their International Partners

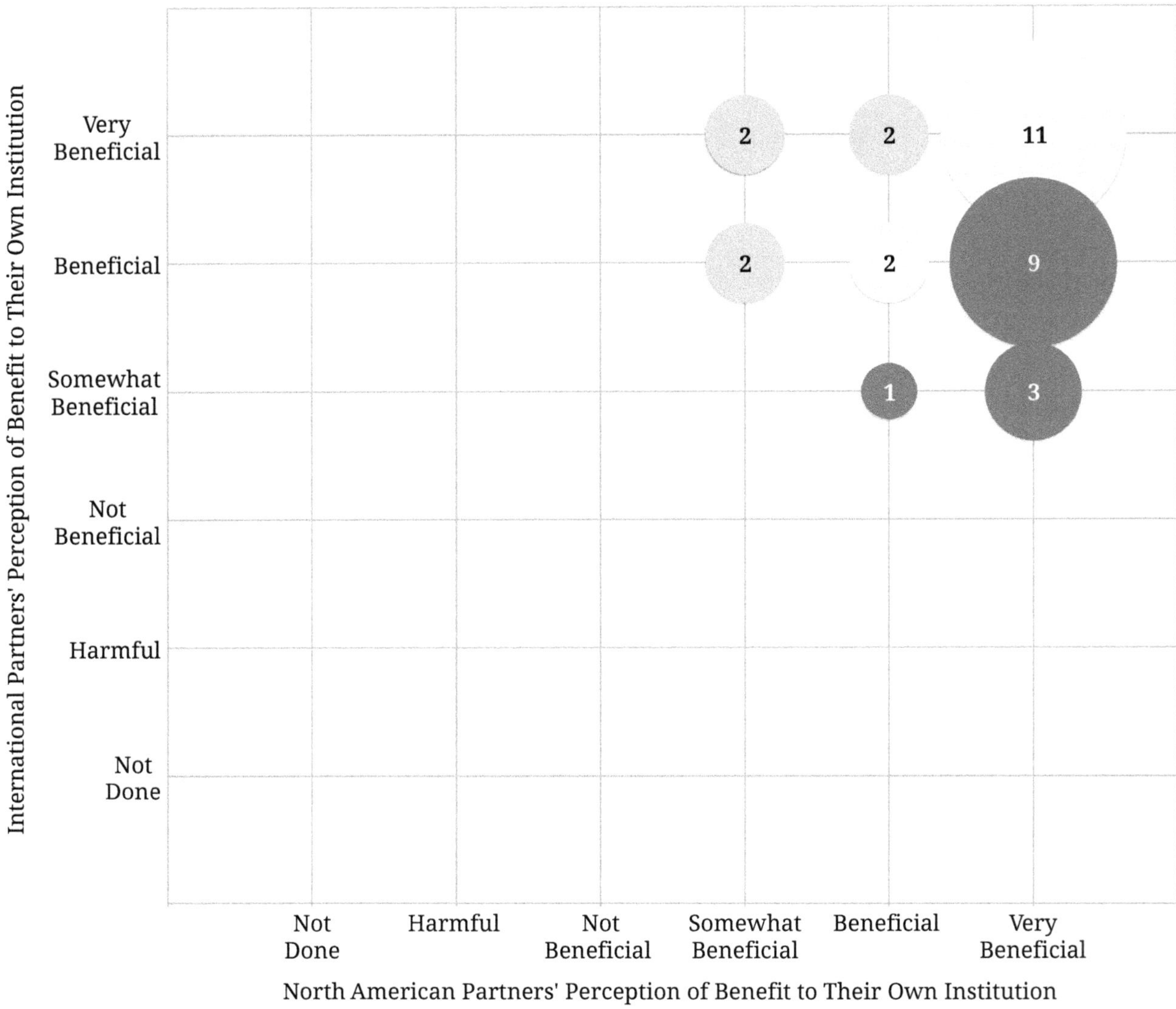

FACTORS CORRELATED WITH PERCEIVED EQUITY AND FULFILLMENT OF NEEDS IN COLLABORATIONS: STATISTICAL ASSESSMENT

Collaboration Assessment

As previously discussed, North American academic institutions and international partners were asked to assess how well they are collaborating with their global health partners as one measure of partnership equity (see the Methods section for a detailed description of included variables, with descriptive statistics presented in Tables 4 and 5). In statistical analyses of survey data (Tables 8 and 9), NAAI funding and the adequacy of North American student training were associated with significantly more favorable assessments by North American academic institutions of how well they were collaborating with their global health partners. Similarly, funding and the adequacy of North American student training were associated with significantly more favorable assessments by international

Figure 26. Comparison of Benefits in Terms of Global Health Impact as Perceived by North American Academic Institutions and as Perceived by their International Partners

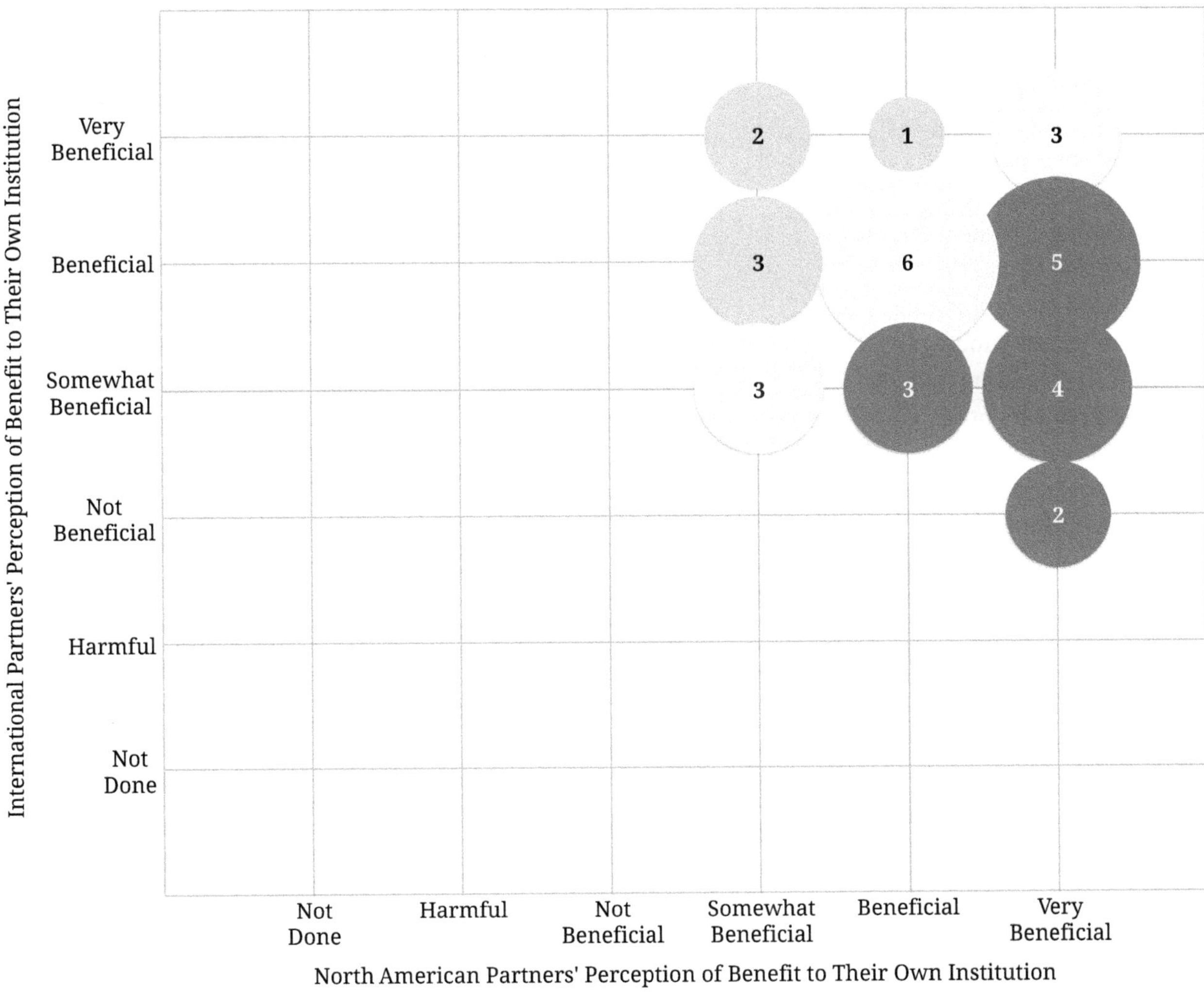

partner respondents. In addition, increases in the collaborative investments (e.g., cash resources, collaborative research grants, student training, provision of advisers for faculty, and/or curriculum development support) that international partners received from North American academic institutions were associated with significantly more favorable assessments of collaborations by international institutions.

Needs Fulfillment

In addition to assessing how well they were collaborating with their North American global health partners, international institutions reported on how well their global health partnerships with North American academic institutions were fulfilling their own institutional needs (Table 10). Our statistical analyses identified several factors associated with a significantly higher level of fulfillment. Funding in general was associated with international institutions reporting their needs as fulfilled, and numerous funding sources (e.g., NIH, UN

Table 8. Factors Associated with North American Academic Institutions' Assessment of Their Collaborations with Global Health Partners

	NAAI Collaborations Scale	
Independent Variables	*Relationship*	*p-value*
NAAI Funding Source	+	**0.05**
University Funding	–	0.9
NIH Funding	+	0.1
PEPFAR Funding	+	0.2
Other Government Funding	+	0.3
External Grants/Contracts	+	0.06
Private Donor Funding	+	0.3
Foundation Funding	+	**0.03**
NAAI NIH Funding Amount	+	0.6
NAAI Endowment	+	0.3
NAAI Private	+	0.3
NAAI Part of Larger Institutional Partnerships	+	0.7
NAAI Enrollment	–	0.4
NAAI Scope of Coursework, Certificate, Major, or Degree Offerings	–	0.7
NAAI Assessment of North American Student Training	+	**<0.001**

Note: Additional information for each variable is outlined in the Methods section.

Table 9. Factors Associated with International Institutions' Assessment of Their Collaborations with North American Partners

	IPI Collaborations Scale	
Independent Variables	*Relationship*	*p-value*
IPI Funding Source	+	0.3
North American University	+	0.4
NIH	+	0.3
PEPFAR	–	0.8
MEPI Funding	–	0.7
Other Government	+	0.5
External Grants/Contracts	+	0.5
UN Agencies	+	0.09
NGO	+	**0.05**
Private Donor	+	0.8
Foundation	+	**0.04**
IPI—Collaborations and Investments Received	+	**0.05**
IPI—Type of Institutions		
Private Academic	–	0.3
NGO	–	0.1
Government Agency	–	0.1
Other Agency	+	0.5
IPI Scope of Coursework, Certificate, Major, or Degree Offerings	+	**0.003**
IPI Assessment of North American Student Training	+	**<0.001**

Note: Additional information for each variable is outlined in the Methods section.

Table 10. Factors Associated with International Institutions' Assessments of How Well Their Partnership Needs Are Fulfilled by Their North American Partners

	IPI Needs Fulfillment Scale	
Independent Variables	*Relationship*	*p-value*
IPI Funding Source	+	**0.03**
North American University	+	0.3
NIH	+	**0.01**
PEPFAR	+	0.9
MEPI Funding	+	0.5
Other Government	+	0.2
External Grants/Contracts	+	0.1
UN Agencies	+	**0.02**
NGO	+	**0.002**
Private Donor	+	0.3
Foundation	+	**0.003**
IPI—Collaborations and Investments Received	+	**0.006**
IPI—Type of Institutions		
Private Academic	+	0.1
NGO	+	0.09
Government Agency	–	0.5
Other Agency	–	0.2
IPI Scope of Coursework, Certificate, Major, or Degree Offerings	+	**0.003**
IPI Assessment of North American Student Training	+	**0.03**
IPI Collaboration Assessment	+	**0.001**

Note: Additional information for each variable is outlined in the Methods section.

agencies, NGO, and Foundation funding) were associated with increases in needs being fulfilled when analyzed individually. In addition, higher amounts of collaborative investments that international institutions received from their North American partners and the international partners' appraisals of how well their collaborations are working were both associated with increased needs fulfillment—suggesting that both the quantity and quality of collaborative engagements with North American universalities are associated with increases in how well international partners' needs are being fulfilled. Finally, more favorable perceptions concerning the adequacy of North American student training were associated with increased fulfillment.

Adequacy and Usefulness of the Collaborative Investments

Perceptions concerning the adequacy of North American student training were positively associated with how well collaborative investments from North American partners met the expectations of international institutions (data not shown). In addition, partnerships rated higher in terms of how well they were collaborating together were associated with higher ratings of how well collaborative investments met the expectations of international partners. These findings suggest that how well international partner's expectations are being met in regards to the collaborative investments they receive has a great deal to do with their perceptions of adequacy of training of North American students and how well they are working with their North American partners. It is interesting to highlight that funding was not significantly associated with how well collaborative investments met the expectations of international institutions.

Reflections

These findings suggest that, in general, global health partnerships are mutually beneficial for both North American academic and international institutions—particularly in areas of education and research and to a lesser degree in positive global health impact. Moreover, a substantial proportion of North American academic and international institutions rate their collaborations as working well and successfully fulfilling the institutional needs of international partners. Given this evidence of successful collaborations between North American academic and international institutions, we now turn to consider potential steps for increasing the sustainability of successful global health programs.

2 Sustainability of Global Health Programs: A Framework for Success

Many of the "inputs" that help create successful academic global health programs[1] are also beneficial for creating, developing, and maintaining strong global health partnerships. To the extent that global health partnerships are vital for successful North American Global Health academic programs (i.e., "you can't do [global health] from a desk" or in isolation), one rubric for gauging the health and vitality of these programs is to assess the sustainability of their global health partnerships.[2]

With this in mind, and with the findings from this study and from a review of the relevant literature, we developed a *Framework for Success* that proposes 10 key components for starting, developing, and sustaining successful global health programs. We anticipate this framework will also favorably position programs to realize success in developing and sustaining global health partnerships. Many of these components were also guided by actions that interview respondents said they had failed to do initially or wish they had done. While explicitly following a chronological order of the 10 building blocks may not always be necessary or feasible, it is likely that some steps should precede others. To summarize, this framework consists of the following components:

1. GAUGE STUDENT AND FACULTY ENTHUSIASM AND SUPPORT, AND IDENTIFY CHAMPIONS AND ORGANIZE A CORE TEAM

Gauging student and faculty enthusiasm for global health may be less important at academic institutions that already have established international health or related programs or departments, but for new or contemplated academic global health programs, student and faculty interest are critical. As many academic institution global health leaders commented in interviews—*it is all about the students.* This was echoed in the case studies. Saba and Brewer (2008), in discussing global health at McGill University, state that "schools should take advantage of students' energy and enthusiasm. There is a large and growing interest among medical students for global health educational programs; they can be essential partners in developing programs, raising awareness, and advocating for change within the

1. Matheson et al., "Sustainability and Growth of University Global Health Programs."
2. Ibid.

Table 11. A Framework for Success in Academic Global Health Programs: 10 Key Components

A Framework for Success
1. Gauge Student and Faculty Enthusiasm and Support, and Identify Champions and Organize a Core Team
2. Prepare a Strategic Plan including Vision and Mission Statements, and Short- and Long-Term Goals
3. Secure Institutional Support and Baseline Funding
4. Establish a Centralized Presence: Program, Center, Institute, Department
5. Develop Future Leaders
6. Guide Student Enthusiasm and Manage Expectations
7. Further Develop Existing Global Health Partnerships and Identify New Partnerships
8. Program Evaluation: Establish and Refine Metrics for Success and Regularly Monitor Progress
9. Develop and Maintain Communication
10. Build Interdisciplinary Networks: Cross-campus, Cross-community, and Internationally

faculty."[3] At McGill, this was manifested in various student-run global health groups that led scholarship programs, organized pre-departure programs to prepare students for international experiences, and organized a simulated World Health Organization (WHO) conference. Often student interest and support are key sources of energy in establishing global health programs. In an interview, one director of a global health program described the importance of structuring global health activities around educational programs that cater to students: "The lifeblood of universities is student interests." Additionally, another university global health leader suggested that programs "engage student interaction whenever possible—lots of students are really interested in global health and you can create win-wins between their educational needs and your needs."

Just as student interest and enthusiasm are vital to build a successful global health program, so are the interest, enthusiasm, and resources of faculty members. Several global health leaders at academic institutions particularly highlighted the importance of global health champions and core faculty teams. Champions can be key faculty members or other academic leaders who are already committed to global health and often already have established global health-related projects and partnerships. The commitment and experience of such champions help provide leadership, commitment, and resolve in setting up program infrastructure, gaining campus-wide support, and identifying potential sources of initial funding. Their drive helps to get ideas off the ground that would otherwise, as an international professor described, "stay just on paper." They can be particularly useful in bridging disciplines where global health efforts have been siloed—such silos could be termed "cylinders of excellence," which are not optimal for engaging global partners in collaborative programs. In a case study of global health at the University of Toronto, where a common concern among faculty was the lack of communication between departments, "many

3. N. Saba and T. F. Brewer, "Beyond Borders: Building Global Health Programs at McGill University Faculty of Medicine," *Academic Medicine* 83, no. 2 (2008): 185–191.

identified the role of individuals acting as facilitators as essential to forming linkages."[4] Ideally, a program will have several global health champions who collaborate in forming a core team of faculty for starting and then developing the global health program at their university and who are especially influential in drafting the program's mission statement.

2. PREPARE A STRATEGIC PLAN INCLUDING VISION AND MISSION STATEMENTS, AND SHORT- AND LONG-TERM GOALS

How global health is to be defined, and once defined, how it is to be organized and implemented are topics of ongoing debate as highlighted in the *Sustainability and Growth of University Global Health Programs* report. This debate is further evident in the extant literature, with one claiming that global health and public health are one in the same,[5] while others perceive it as a distinct discipline or a more interdisciplinary field.[6, 7, 8, 9, 10, 11] While debate continues concerning a universal definition for global health, it is important that individual academic institution global health programs establish mission statements that clearly define what the mission of global health means for their program and what they see as their contribution to global health as an academic discipline and as a broader field. As an indication of the importance of preparing mission statements early on when establishing a global health program, of the 15 articles (Appendix F) identified in our literature review as case studies for establishing a global health program, the subjects most frequently presented were the various programs' mission statements and/or accompanying short- and long-term goals and how these steps set the tone and direction for developing the related programs. For example, the Emory Global Health Institute's primary goals are to develop a strong academic and research infrastructure, pursue and maintain global partnerships, and promote interdisciplinary global health work on campus.[12] These broad goals speak to the vision of Emory's breadth, depth, and resources in global health. Alternatively, goals may be more focused to reflect more focused activities. The Mount Sinai Global Health Residency Track has the goal to "provide participants with a foundation in global health issues and population-based health care, a chance to develop basic research and public health skills in the field, and the opportunity to build professional relationships for future career development."[13] Goals will inform specific activities, so it is important to think of whether current or future capacity is reflected within a stated mission.

---

4. A. D. Pinto et al., "A case study of global health at the university: implications for research and action," *Global Health Action* 7 (2014): 24526.
5. L. P. Fried et al., "Global health is public health," *Lancet* 375 (2010): 535–537.
6. Koplan et al., "Towards a Common Definition of Global Health."
7. Beaglehole and Bonita, "What Is Global Health?"
8. Rowson et al., "Conceptualising Global Health: Theoretical Issues and Their Relevance for Teaching."
9. M. Morse, "Responsible Global Health Engagement: A Road Map to Equity for Academic Partnerships," *Journal of Graduate Medical Education* 6, no. 2 (2014): 347–348.
10. Olapade-Olaopa et al., "Growing Partnerships: Leveraging the Power of Collaboration Through the Medical Education Partnership Initiative."
11. Anderson et al., "Creating a Charter of Collaboration for International University Partnerships: The Elmina Declaration for Human Resources for Health."
12. J. P Koplan and R. L. Baggett, "The Emory Global Health Institute: Developing Partnerships to Improve Health Through Research, Training, and Service," *Academic Medicine* 83, no. 2 (2008): 128–133.
13. N. Anandaraja et al., "The Design and Implementation of a Multidisciplinary Global Health Residency Track at the Mount Sinai School of Medicine," *Academic Medicine* 83, no. 10 (2008): 924–928.

Table 12. Phases in Business and Organizational Development

Phase	*Main Activities*	*Results*
1. Starting Up	• Develop vision into a real plan • Obtain initial funding/financing • Set up organizational structure • Initiate partnerships	• High motivation • Officially established • Initial products realized
2. Consolidation	• Maintain personnel, increase production • Streamline operations • Solidify partnerships	• Efficient structures • Good staff • All costs covered • Reliable partnerships
3. Expansion	• Increase personnel, but maintain focus • Emphasize quality	• Organization operating successfully • Capitalize on success
4. Diversification	• Maintain personnel, but diversify focus • Diversify activities	• Fixed costs covered by several activities

With a mission statement in place, new academic programs should set short- and long-term goals. This process may benefit from a study of business and organizational development models. One such model[14] depicts four phases in business or organization development and is adapted and summarized in Table 12.

These phases suggest that it is advisable to initially concentrate on a few key areas as the global health program grows. This suggestion was echoed by many of the academic institution global health leaders who advised that it will be difficult for younger programs to do a wide variety of activities from the beginning and to do them all well. Younger programs are more likely to realize success if they have specific areas of focus, such as HIV/AIDS, MNCH, or neglected tropical diseases, and engage partnerships in specific geographies. This is particularly the case for areas of focus and a caution for geographies that are already inundated by established programs.

3. SECURE INSTITUTIONAL SUPPORT AND BASELINE FUNDING

The importance of support from nonfaculty institutional stakeholders, both financial and otherwise, was described by many academic institution global health leaders. Financially, institutional support was deemed essential most frequently among North American survey respondents. Successful programs also have strong leadership support at multiple levels. In forming global health programs, nearly all published case studies reviewed cited buy-in from deans or other leaders as an important initial step. In forming a Global Health Residency Track, each faculty member within the Global Health Center at Mount Sinai met with

14. "Planning and Managing Your Business," Organic Business Guide, accessed August 26, 2015, https://en.wikibooks.org/wiki/Organic_Business_Guide/Planning_and_managing_your_business#Management_structures_and_capacity.

the chairperson in their respective department to gain support.[15] Such support helps to maintain effective programs and partnerships.

Institutional support is important even from seemingly unrelated areas of campus. One office of global health described maintaining a standing monthly meeting with their institution's legal counsel, which is particularly useful in navigating policies and regulations surrounding foreign students coming to the United States and for operating in other countries. Others cited working closely with Internal Review Boards and Offices of Sponsored Programs (e.g., for managing grants and contracts) as key stakeholders. Above all, Risk Management offices were frequently referenced, both as an important on-campus stakeholder to involve, and as a source of challenge and frustration when trying to establish and maintain partnerships in less secure areas. Many North American interview respondents described the importance of communicating with these offices, both to explain and advocate for the importance of their international programs and to better understand risks involved for their students. To integrate risk management among multiple stakeholders, the University of Wisconsin–Madison enlisted a committee of 24 faculty and staff members across units and divisions to identify policies around risk management when developing their center.[16] Overall, securing institutional support at all levels is a way to tap expertise in various aspects of program management and ensure adherence to institutional policies. However, in this regard, one Department Chair said that ". . . it is not all just about compliance with existing rules and regulations; it is about adapting to new settings and situations, and providing new types of support for global health programs."

Baseline funding was the most consistently referenced challenge reported by both survey and interview respondents. The interviews and the published case studies identified a variety of approaches to identifying funding. Some programs, such as the University of Washington Department of Global Health and the Emory Global Health Institute, were started through substantial funds from either external or internal sources (in these cases foundation funding and university start-up funds).[17, 18] However, several successful academic institution global health leaders indicated that start-up funds were initially modest. The Global Health Curriculum at Weill Cornell Medical College operated for its first two years on a "modest budget, covered by informal cost sharing between the three offices that are stakeholders in the program." Later, this was formalized so that each office contributed to program costs up to $10,000 per year, and additional support came from the dean and various internal offices.[19] For the Center for Global Health at University of Wisconsin–

15. See Anandaraja, "The Design and Implementation of a Multidisciplinary Global Health Residency Track at the Mount Sinai School of Medicine."

16. C. Haq et al., "Creating a Center for Global Health at the University of Wisconsin–Madison," *Academic Medicine* 83, no. 2 (2008): 148–153.

17. F. B. Stapleton et al., "Addressing Global Health Through the Marriage of Public Health and Medicine: Developing the University of Washington Department of Global Health," *Academic Medicine* 81, no. 10 (2006): 897–901.

18. See Koplan and Baggett, "The Emory Global Health Institute."

19. E. R. Francis et al., "The Global Health Curriculum of Weill Cornell Medical College: How One School Developed a Global Health Program," *Academic Medicine* 87, no. 9 (2012): 1296–1302.

Madison, support from deans was complemented by mobilization of alumni to solicit donations.[20] This speaks to the importance of diverse funding sources. Once a secure, stable funding base is established, many programs have continued to expand and diversify their portfolios, as diversified types and sources of funding brought unique opportunities as to how they can be used to create stability over time.

4. ESTABLISH A CENTRALIZED PRESENCE (PROGRAM, CENTER, INSTITUTE, DEPARTMENT)

An important step, cited in the literature and also discussed by interview respondents, for program success is the potential benefit of centralization. Centralization helps facilitate coordination among various stakeholders on campus, in the local community, and between global health partners. Coordination contributes to efficiencies, including efficient dissemination of information to students and faculty who are interested in global health curriculum, research, or applied activities. A centralized presence is essential in establishing institution-wide policies, guidelines, and standardized processes for global operations. In the literature reviewed, the impetus for (and benefit of) creating a centralized presence was often to bring together the global health work being implemented among different components of the health sciences.[21, 22, 23] A centralized global health body can also "facilitate major institutional bridges between the health sciences and the rest of campus,"[24] encouraging interdisciplinary collaborations and a greater understanding of global health across communities. Beyond intra-institutional centralization within the academic institution, inter-institutional coordination and creation of institutional networks is facilitated by bodies such as CUGH, which provide a platform for communication and organization among institutions pursuing global health work.

There are logistic considerations in centralizing global health presence. In establishing a centralized presence on campus, sufficient administrative support is essential. Several interview respondents reported that funding for administrative staff must be considered early on in the development of a global health program. As another university global health leader concisely asserted, "Have adequate resources for administrative infrastructure; 20 percent time will not work!" A strong administrative component to a global health program confers many benefits: it can create a central repository of all global health activities,[25] and collaborative agreements, and can help program sustainability.[26]

---

20. See Haq, "Creating a Center for Global Health at the University of Wisconsin–Madison."
21. See Koplan and Baggett, "The Emory Global Health Institute."
22. T. C. Quinn, "The Johns Hopkins Center for Global Health: Transcending Borders for World Health," *Academic Medicine* 83, no. 2 (2008): 134–142.
23. See Haq, "Creating a Center for Global Health at the University of Wisconsin–Madison."
24. Ibid.
25. See Saba and Brewer, "Beyond Borders: Building Global Health Programs at McGill University Faculty of Medicine."
26. See Francis, "The Global Health Curriculum of Weill Cornell Medical College."

5. DEVELOP FUTURE LEADERS

Development and sustainability of this emerging field requires ongoing identification and development of new leadership and champions. As one global health program director explained, it is important to find "people who really get the vision easily, are quick learners, and are not encrusted in historic calcification and are ready to think outside the box." In discussing strategies for sustainability, another U.S. dean explained how global health leaders must model the type of behavior they expect students to follow, both in terms of research integrity and interpersonal skills and the effects this can have even decades into the future. The same holds true for international students trained in North America; through mechanisms such as the NIH Fogarty International Center and the Afya Bora Consortium Fellowship, these students are able to train in North America and return to leadership positions in their countries of origin.

6. GUIDE STUDENT ENTHUSIASM AND MANAGE EXPECTATIONS

While student enthusiasm and altruism are vital for creating energy within academic global health programs, students' needs and interests can also be a source of challenge and frustration. Most interview respondents in North America cited an explicit desire to avoid the "medical tourism" model. Even in research- and education-focused trips, several respondents described situations in which student priorities conflicted with greater partnership goals. Many graduate or health profession students enter programs with a range of international experiences, along with often very specific geographic interests and goals that can be difficult to manage. One respondent explained, "Geographic areas wax and wane in popularity; whereas many students in the past only wanted to go to Africa, now they're more interested in South America or Southeast Asia." Graduate students often prefer traveling on their own as well, which can be logistically more challenging than integrated student programs. The dean of another public health program echoed this finding, citing the desire of many students to do independent study rather than utilize existing partnerships, resulting in a situation where "it wasn't entirely clear that they were getting all the supervision that they needed." This program has since developed a strategy in which student applications are carefully scrutinized in order to "manage trainees and students in a way that doesn't bring more disruption to [the] international partner's system." We strongly concur with this approach. Student expectations can also create a challenge for international hosting institutions. For example, several international respondents, in both surveys and interviews, described situations in which they did not feel that North American students possessed the requisite language or cultural competency to work in their low-resource setting, or they felt that the lower capacities in their country did not meet the North American students' expectations.

7. FURTHER DEVELOP EXISTING GLOBAL HEALTH PARTNERSHIPS AND IDENTIFY NEW PARTNERSHIPS

Global health partnerships are critical to the success and vitality of global health programs not overloaded with other existing partnerships.[27] New or recently established programs

27. Rosenberg et al., *Real Collaborations: What It Takes for Global Health to Succeed.*

may benefit from relationships and projects that were already established by faculty members on campus, but that had yet to be organized into a unified program. This was the most common strategy described by academic institution global health leaders.

Young programs may be dismayed to realize that many potential international partners are already inundated by other, more established programs seeking to create or maintain collaborative relationships. In our survey, certain (primarily English-speaking) countries were disproportionately represented as partners for North American institutions. One interviewee described the "partner noise" created by multiple foreign organizations doing work in the same small East African community.

Over 50 percent of the global health partnerships reported by international institutional respondents in our survey were with institutions outside of North America. Moreover, even though 97 percent of international partners reported that South-North partnerships had been the most valuable in the past (Figure 27a), only 61 percent reported that developing South-North partnerships would be their highest priority moving forward (Figure 27b). Given these current priorities, one global health leader at a North American institution remarked, "This may necessitate creativity and flexibility on the part of younger programs as they may need to start out in newer or uniquely innovative areas of focus and/or geographies." A leader at an international university with many North American and regional partnerships explained that "both types of relationships are quite important. We want to keep having these North to South relationships, but they are not exclusive. We need to create better networks with countries in the region. [However] we still need to learn how to work better with collaborators in the North."

Figure 27a. Global Health Partnerships: Historically Most Valuable

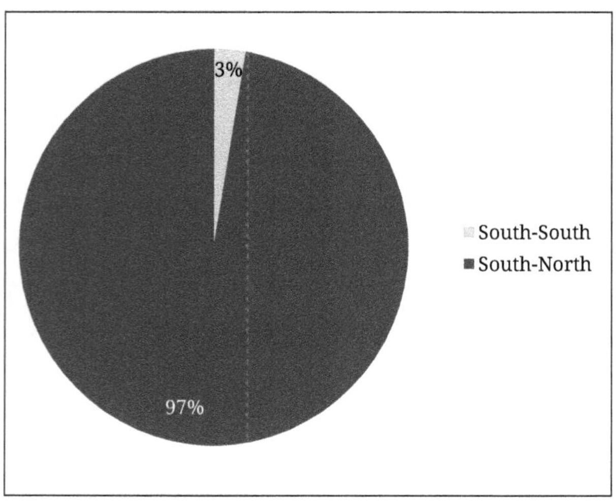

Figure 27b. Global Health Partnerships: Priority for Future Collaborations

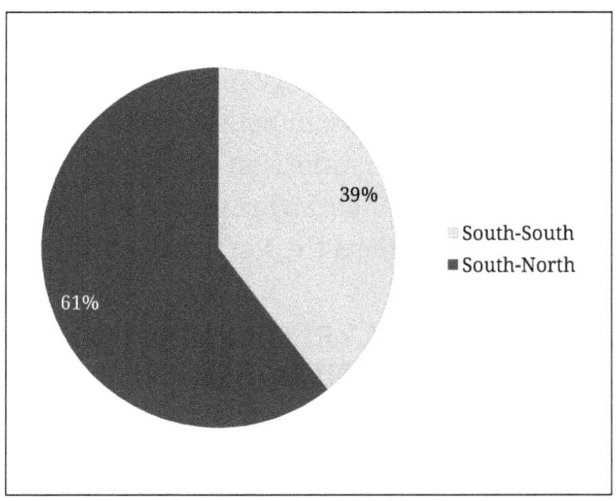

8. PROGRAM EVALUATION: ESTABLISH AND REFINE METRICS FOR SUCCESS AND REGULARLY MONITOR PROGRESS

Once global health programs and partnerships are in operation, it is important to define, monitor, and evaluate success. In discussing monitoring and evaluation mechanisms with North American and international global health leaders, it was apparent that current implementation of evaluation ranged from nonexistent to informal to formal. Establishing and refining evaluation metrics is an important step in creating a sustainable global health program. In the case studies reviewed, there were many suggestions of possible metrics. Haq et al. (2008) lists outcome measures for the University of Wisconsin–Madison Center for Global Health in four categories: educational; research; partnerships, service projects, and exchanges; and administrative. Examples of outcomes in each category, respectively, include number and location of global health courses and field experiences, number and type of global health research projects, health outcomes for target populations (before and after interventions), and assessment of program and activities by participating units.[28] In the Mount Sinai Global Health Residency Track, impact is measured through online and in-class evaluations as well as focus groups.[29] Although developing metrics can be challenging, given the breadth of global health programs, leaders concur that it is worth doing.[30, 31]

9. DEVELOP AND MAINTAIN COMMUNICATION

Communication is essential in every aspect of starting and developing global health programs and related partnerships. Personal relationships are the foundation for good communication. Current technology allows people to "be in quick, rapid, and inexpensive communication with people all over the world,"[32] and many programs have leveraged this capability to improve communication internally and with external partners. Distance learning, webinars, and web-based programs may all be utilized to this effect.[33] Throughout interviews conducted with global health leaders, several cited personal relationships as central to successful communication and noted that lack of communication is a pitfall to be avoided. To maintain these relationships, regular conversations and site visits or other face-to-face interactions are important. As one global health leader described it, successful partnerships are "founded on the integrity of interpersonal relationships with mutual goals."

---

28. See Haq, "Creating a Center for Global Health at the University of Wisconsin–Madison."

29. See Anandaraja, "The Design and Implementation of a Multidisciplinary Global Health Residency Track at the Mount Sinai School of Medicine."

30. See Koplan and Baggett, "The Emory Global Health Institute."

31. D. Ozgediz et al., "Surgical Training and Global Health Initial Results of a 5-Year Partnership with a Surgical Training Program in a Low-Income Country," *Archives of Surgery* 143, no. 9 (2008): 860–865.

32. H. T. Debas and T. J. Coates. "The University of California Global Health Institute Opportunities and Challenges," *Infectious Disease Clinics of North America* 25 (2011): 499–509.

33. S. H. Vermund et al., "Building Global Health Through a Center-Without-Walls: The Vanderbilt Institute for Global Health," *Academic Medicine* 83, no. 2 (2008): 154–164.

10. BUILD INTERDISCIPLINARY NETWORKS: CROSS-CAMPUS, CROSS-COMMUNITY, AND INTERNATIONALLY

A key characteristic of academic global health is that it recognizes the need for an interdisciplinary approach. Recognizing the strengths to be gained through developing interdisciplinary networks, many schools with established global health programs have sought to attract additional faculty and partners through building relationships across campus and their broader communities. Of the 15 articles reviewed, 11 described their programs as "interdisciplinary," and having at least one interdisciplinary program is a requirement for membership in CUGH. The University of California Global Health Institute is one example of an academic global health model that seeks to integrate global health efforts across multiple institutions as it has created a "transdisciplinary, multi-campus academic global health model" that links 10 campuses across California.[34] Social sciences, business, engineering, and public policy were some of the many disciplines mentioned for collaboration. Interdisciplinary work also encompasses partnerships with local communities as well as internationally. At the University of California, San Francisco (UCSF), the motto for global health work is "think globally, act locally, and collaborate internationally."[35] The Duke Global Health Institute was formed with the support of a campus-wide committee and is not housed in one school, instead functioning as a university-wide institute. It is also important to note that building an interdisciplinary network is facilitated by an academic environment; this is one advantage that academic institutions hold over nonprofits and government agencies in their pursuit of global health.

Reflections

The steps identified in this roadmap will require time for development; many cannot be readily undertaken or achieved simultaneously, but most of these steps need to be established and in operation to move forward. Likewise, successful, equitable partnerships take time to develop. Communication is key, and establishing effective metrics of evaluation that assess the needs and accomplishments of both partners and that help the partnership operate in a mutually beneficial manner is an iterative process that will take time to establish and refine.

Discussion

Overall, the most consistent factor related to the overall success and sustainability of academic global health programs and partnerships identified in our research is *time* (i.e., the duration of the partnership). Start-up businesses often take five to six years to become fully established,[36] and start-up academic global health programs similarly will require

34. See Debas and Coates, "The University of California Global Health Institute Opportunities and Challenges."

35. S. B. Macfarlane, "Think Globally, Act Locally, and Collaborate Internationally: Global Health Sciences at the University of California, San Francisco" *Academic Medicine* 83, no. 2 (2008): 173–179.

36. "Planning and Managing Your Business," Organic Business Guide.

time to develop and mature, especially when they rely on strong global health partnerships as a key component of their long-term success. Global health impact can take even longer. In a study in the United Kingdom, the time lag between research expenditure and health benefits was estimated at 15 years.[37] These benefits can take the form of health system cost savings, a healthy workforce, and overall societal and economic gains.[38] As one might expect, the time lag in benefits will vary by country, project, and setting.

Another interesting thread throughout this study was the evolving dynamics of North-South and South-South collaborations in the field of global health. There are also, however, increasing collaborations and partnerships *among* academic institutions in the global North. An example of this is the NIH Global Health Program for Fellows and Scholars, which is comprised of five consortia, each involving four universities, each of which partners with six or more low- and middle-income countries. This program promotes collaboration among U.S. academic institutions and decreases competition in the field, suggesting that partnerships in North America can be encouraged as well.

Finally, it will be interesting to observe the extent to which global health continues to proliferate across North America. CUGH lists 157 North American academic institutions with global health programs in its 2013 Global Health Programs Database. However, with over 2,900 postsecondary Title IV institutions granting four-year degrees in the United States alone,[39] this leaves many more institutions that could potentially develop some level of global health programming.

STRENGTHS

To our knowledge, no survey of this kind has been done before. As a groundbreaking investigation of global health partnerships, this study benefits from the mixed methods design, which used quantitative surveys and in-depth qualitative interviews, as well as a review of published case studies on global health programs at North American academic institutions. The high (81.2 percent) survey response rate among CUGH members indicates that the data are highly representative of North American CUGH-member institutions. In addition, the high survey response rate (75.8 percent) among international partner institutions, as well as the 11 key informant interviews with global health leaders from international partner institutions, suggest that our findings also provide substantial insight to the perspectives of international partners.

LIMITATIONS

Although we initially approached 20 non-CUGH member institutions with global health programs in our survey, the response rate was so low (three) as to render any information about these institutions or comparison to CUGH counterparts inconclusive. The lack of

37. Health Economics Research Group, *Medical Research: What's it worth?* (2008): 7.
38. Ibid.
39. U.S. Department of Education, National Center for Education Statistics. *Digest of Education Statistics, 2013* (NCES 2015-011), Table 105.50, May 2015; http://nces.ed.gov/pubs2015/2015011.pdf.

non-CUGH institution perspective may mean that important information about how smaller or new global health programs function was left out of our research. For international institutions, the sample selection strategy (international institutions were identified through North American partners and may not be representative of partner institution experience more broadly), the distribution of survey participants (43 percent from partnerships identified by North American institutions as "high performing," 40 percent from "middle standing," and 17 percent from "struggling"), and survey attrition (some respondents did not complete the entire survey, which led to smaller numbers of responses for some questions) may have introduced selection bias, despite efforts taken by the research team to avoid such bias. Furthermore, the survey was distributed in English only, which may have limited responses from non-English-speaking partners.

Finally, responses on behalf of institutions do at some level reflect the experiences and perceptions of the individuals providing them as well as their cultural background, and it is unlikely that any individual understands all goals, offerings, and priorities of their institution perfectly. Many of the important aspects of these partnerships (e.g., equity, impact and benefits) are concepts that don't have well-characterized metrics from which to evaluate success and hence were assessed by self-reporting of perceptions of these factors within partnerships. Therefore personal bias is a potential weakness of this survey, as there is no guarantee responses cover all facets of the programs they report on. Moreover, respondents from both North American academic and international partnering institutions may have felt obligated to respond more favorably to survey and interview questions in order to provide a positive depiction of their programs and partnerships, despite assurances that individual responses would remain anonymous.

Conclusions

The success of development and sustainability of global health programs shares many criteria in common with the success of development and sustainability of mutually beneficial and equitable global health partnerships. Recognition that funding is vital to both of these endeavors is not surprising; both programs and partnerships typically require substantial seed funding to get started. Such funding must be continually cultivated and diversified to enable programs and partnerships to develop and flourish. Financial resources can be a challenge; tuition revenues alone are often inadequate to support global health programs, and students frequently help pay for their own international experiences. Given the evidence presented suggesting that global health programs and partnerships are realizing positive benefits, it behooves academic institutions and funding organizations (e.g., the Clinton Foundation, CIDA, the Gates Foundation, IDRC, NIH, USAID, CDC, and UN agencies) to further their support of these programs and partnerships. Success, however, also requires more than financial resources.

The findings presented in this study provide evidence that global health partnerships are mutually beneficial to North American academic and partnering international institutions. These benefits are greatest for education and research collaborations, but partnerships are also beneficial for achieving global health impact. North American academic institutions are somewhat more positive in their overall assessment of benefits derived, both for themselves and for their international partners, but international institutions report high levels of satisfaction with the benefits and equity of collaborative investments they are receiving from their North American partners.

The demographic composition of global health partnerships is rapidly changing. International institutions actively engage with numerous global partners outside of North America; while the vast majority cited South-North collaborations as the most valuable to date, the fact that nearly 40 percent say that developing South-South collaborations will be their highest priority in the future is of interest. One international interviewee described South-South collaborations as "horizontal collaborations" as opposed to North-South vertical collaborations. Many North American academic institutions are also expanding their networks of affiliation beyond their local campuses to partner with other North American and European academic institutions. We interpret these changes as efforts by both international institutions and North American academic institutions to diversify their partnerships. Future research should confirm and explore the reasons for such a shift in partnership priorities.

The importance of funding for program and partnership success was universal among survey and interview respondents, but it is just one of multiple factors identified. Institutional and leadership support, personal relationships, champions, student enthusiasm, effective communication, and time are all important considerations. Students in particular are a great resource and source of energy in North American global health programs. However, their needs and expectations must be well managed.

Many global health partnerships have lacked formal evaluation. This fact, and the diversity of partnerships, makes it difficult to draw firm conclusions on how partnerships function and to make comparisons across partnerships. However, we hope this study offers some clarity to this topic as well as points to consider for North American and international institutions seeking to establish, maintain, or improve their partnerships to better address global health.

Appendix A. North American Academic Institution Survey Letter and Instrument

Introduction

In May 2014, the Center for Strategic and International Studies (CSIS) published a report with the University of Washington and the Consortium of Universities for Global Health (CUGH) that examined the sustainability and growth of global health programs in U.S. and Canadian universities. Most university stakeholders cited strong international partnerships as critical to the success and sustainability of their efforts.[1]

Effective collaborations between partners involve the mutual development of goals, planning, implementation, and evaluation of performance and benefits. The rapidly growing interest in global health training, service, and research activities at universities has given way to a surge in international partnerships which stand to benefit from a timely assessment of how well these partnerships are working and how they can be improved to maximize synergy and mutual benefits.

The University of Washington, in collaboration with CUGH and CSIS, is conducting a follow-up study to appraise how well international partnerships are mutually benefiting North American universities and their international partners, including determinants of equity, benefit, harm, sustainability, and to assess the global health impact of these partnerships.

Your response to this survey is being sought to help identify characteristics of success and challenges in relation to international partnerships that need to be overcome in order to have a greater impact on global health. Our goal is to contribute to a better understanding of what is working well, what remains a challenge, and what can be done to improve international partnerships in university global health programs. Your responses will remain anonymous and no university will be linked to your description of partnerships. If you agree, we would like to recognize you for your participation in the study. The results

1. To view the report, see http://csis.org/files/publication/140507_Matheson_UniversityEngagement_Web.pdf.

will be published in collaboration with CUGH and CSIS, and presented to universities engaged in global health.

Thank you in advance for participating in this survey!

Participant Contact Information

1) What is your name?
2) What is the name of your educational institution?
3) What is your title or position?
4) What responsibilities do you have for global health?
5) What is your e-mail address?
6) What is your phone number?

General Information

7) What is the name or names of the principal entity or entities (e.g., department, program, center, institute, etc.) that focus on global health at your institution?
8) Which of the following degrees and programs are offered by your institution and have substantial global health components? Please check all that apply.

   - ☐ One or more global health courses
   - ☐ Certificate
   - ☐ Undergraduate minor
   - ☐ Undergraduate major
   - ☐ Dual or joint undergraduate major
   - ☐ MPH
   - ☐ Masters (non-MPH)
   - ☐ Doctoral (e.g., PhD, DrPH, etc.)
   - ☐ Joint PhD
   - ☐ Health professional (e.g., nursing, vet, medical)
   - ☐ Postgraduate (e.g., fellowships, residency)

- ☐ Dual or joint graduate degree
- ☐ Joint degree between low- and high-income countries
- ☐ Other

9) If "other" is selected above, please specify the degree type:

PART ONE—General Partnership Information

10) In what types of global health partnerships is your institution engaged? *Please check all that apply.*
    - ☐ Medical professional education and/or training
    - ☐ Other health professional education or training (e.g., nursing, public health, social work, pharmacy, dentistry)
    - ☐ Collaborative research
    - ☐ Interventions or services
    - ☐ Health systems development/capacity building
    - ☐ Technology exchange
    - ☐ Policy development & advocacy
    - ☐ Learning and practicum experience for North American students
    - ☐ Learning and practicum experience for international students
    - ☐ Other
    - ☐ We do not have any international global health partnerships
11) If "other" is selected above, please specify the type of global health partnership:
12) If your global health program does not have international partnerships is it interested in developing global health partnerships and what have been the barriers to developing such partnerships?
13) Are your global health partnerships part of larger institutional or university partnerships?
    - ☐ Yes
    - ☐ No
14) If yes, please describe how your global health partnerships fit into larger institutional or university partnerships.

15) On a scale of 1 to 5, please indicate the degree of importance of different sources of funding that are currently received by your institution and used to finance global health partnerships. Please check one box per row.

	Do not receive	*(1) Not important*	*(2) Low importance*	*(3) Medium importance*	*(4) High importance*	*(5) Essential*
University funding	☐	☐	☐	☐	☐	☐
NIH funding (e.g., Fogarty grants, research grants)	☐	☐	☐	☐	☐	☐
PEPFAR (HIV/AIDS related funding)	☐	☐	☐	☐	☐	☐
Other federal government funding (e.g., CDC, USAID, etc.)	☐	☐	☐	☐	☐	☐
Nonfederal government funding/other external grants or contracts	☐	☐	☐	☐	☐	☐
Private donors	☐	☐	☐	☐	☐	☐
Foundations	☐	☐	☐	☐	☐	☐

16) Comments:

17) On a scale of 1 to 5, what is your assessment of the degree of adequacy of the following types of training or orientation provided to students from your institution participating in international global health partnerships? Please check one box per row.

	Is not provided	*(1) Very inadequate*	*(2) Somewhat inadequate*	*(3) Somewhat adequate*	*(4) Adequate*	*(5) Very adequate*
Ethics	□	□	□	□	□	□
Host-country institutional requirements for visitors	□	□	□	□	□	□
Sociocultural aspects of life in the host country	□	□	□	□	□	□
Cultural awareness for engaging in international health work	□	□	□	□	□	□
Language training	□	□	□	□	□	□
Student's role, scope of tasks, and supervision while abroad	□	□	□	□	□	□
Preparation for the challenges of providing care or working in under-resourced settings	□	□	□	□	□	□

18) Comments:

19) On a scale of 1 to 5, please indicate the extent to which international partnerships are beneficial for your global health program in the following areas. Please check one box per row.

	(1) Harmful	*(2) Not beneficial*	*(3) Somewhat beneficial*	*(4) Beneficial*	*(5) Very beneficial*
Student/trainee knowledge acquisition	☐	☐	☐	☐	☐
Attract prospective students, trainees & faculty	☐	☐	☐	☐	☐
Collaborative research	☐	☐	☐	☐	☐
Build student foundations for a career oriented toward global health	☐	☐	☐	☐	☐
Develop leadership	☐	☐	☐	☐	☐
Diversify revenue for the university	☐	☐	☐	☐	☐
Maximize global health impact	☐	☐	☐	☐	☐

20) Are there other benefits for your global health program not listed above?

21) On a scale of 1 to 5, please indicate the extent to which you perceive the following are key benefits of your institution's international partnerships for your international partners. Please check one box per row.

	(1) Harmful	*(2) Not beneficial*	*(3) Somewhat beneficial*	*(4) Beneficial*	*(5) Very beneficial*
Knowledge acquisition	☐	☐	☐	☐	☐
Financial support	☐	☐	☐	☐	☐
Collaborative research	☐	☐	☐	☐	☐

(continued)

	(1) Harmful	(2) Not beneficial	(3) Somewhat beneficial	(4) Beneficial	(5) Very beneficial
Training & mentoring	□	□	□	□	□
Health systems strengthening	□	□	□	□	□
Reciprocal student exchanges, education, training	□	□	□	□	□
Developing leadership	□	□	□	□	□
Beneficial local impact on health	□	□	□	□	□

22) Are there other perceived benefits for your international partners not listed above?

23) On a scale of 1 to 5, please indicate the extent to which your institution's various global health partnerships have developed and evolved in a manner that is mutually beneficial to your university and its international partners. Please check one box per row.

	Not done	*(1) Entirely from your institution's perspective*	*(2) Mostly from your institution's perspective*	*(3) Equally developed*	*(4) Mostly from your international partners' perspectives*	*(5) Entirely from your international partners' perspectives*
Health professional education and/or training	□	□	□	□	□	□
Collaborative research	□	□	□	□	□	□
Interventions or services	□	□	□	□	□	□
Health systems development/ capacity building	□	□	□	□	□	□
Technology exchange	□	□	□	□	□	□

	Not done	(1) Entirely from your institution's perspective	(2) Mostly from your institution's perspective	(3) Equally developed	(4) Mostly from your international partners' perspectives	(5) Entirely from your international partners' perspectives
Policy development & advocacy	☐	☐	☐	☐	☐	☐
Learning and practicum experience for North American students	☐	☐	☐	☐	☐	☐
Learning and practicum experience for international students	☐	☐	☐	☐	☐	☐

24) Comments:

25) On a scale of 1 to 5, please rate how well your global health program is working together with its international partners in the following areas. Please check one box per row.

	Not done	(1) Poor	(2) Fair	(3) Well	(4) Very well	(5) Excellent
Assessing the needs of your international partners	☐	☐	☐	☐	☐	☐
Establishing mutual goals	☐	☐	☐	☐	☐	☐
Addressing the needs of your international partners	☐	☐	☐	☐	☐	☐
Planning, monitoring & evaluating the impact of collaborations	☐	☐	☐	☐	☐	☐
Soliciting & incorporating feedback from your students, faculty & administrative leaders	☐	☐	☐	☐	☐	☐

	Not done	*(1) Poor*	*(2) Fair*	*(3) Well*	*(4) Very well*	*(5) Excellent*
Soliciting and assessing feedback from your university's international partners	□	□	□	□	□	□

26) Comments:

27) What is the most important factor lacking in your current global health partnerships and what can be done to address what is lacking?

28) What is the most exciting new opportunity for your partnerships and how do you think your institution's partnerships can best address this new opportunity?

Part Two

In this section you will be asked to nominate 2–3 international partners that we may contact to participate in the International Partners Survey. In order to represent a wide variety of partnerships we ask that, if possible, you choose partnerships that differ from one another with regards to the type of partnership, implementation duration, and performance.

The following pages are structured so that you will be asked first to provide contact information for a high-performing partnership, second for a middle-standing partnership, and third for a struggling partnership.

PARTNER NUMBER ONE: (HIGH-PERFORMING PARTNERSHIP)

29) Name of academic institution, NGO, other (specify):

30) Country:

31) Name of partnership program (if applicable):

32) Partner classification:

    - □ Public academic institution
    - □ Private academic institution
    - □ Nongovernmental organization
    - □ Other

33) Type of partnership:

- □ Medical professional trainee program
- □ Collaborative research
- □ Health systems development/capacity building
- □ Learning & practicum experience
- □ Other

34) If "other" please specify the type of partnership:

35) Partnership duration:

36) Name of in-country representative:

37) E-mail of in-country representative:

38) Phone number of in-country representative:

39) Name of second in-country representative:

40) E-mail of second in-country representative:

41) Phone number of second in-country representative:

PARTNER NUMBER TWO: (MIDDLE-STANDING PARTNERSHIP)

42) Name of academic institution, NGO, other (specify):

43) Country:

44) Name of partnership program (if applicable):

45) Partner classification:

- □ Public academic institution
- □ Private academic institution
- □ Nongovernmental organization
- □ Other

46) Type of partnership:

- □ Medical professional trainee program
- □ Collaborative research
- □ Health systems development/capacity building

- □ Learning & practicum experience
- □ Other

47) If "other" please specify the type of partnership:
48) Partnership duration:
49) Name of in-country representative:
50) E-mail of in-country representative:
51) Phone number of in-country representative:
52) Name of second in-country representative:
53) E-mail of second in-country representative:
54) Phone number of second in-country representative:

PARTNER NUMBER THREE: (STRUGGLING PARTNERSHIP)

55) Name of academic institution, NGO, other (specify):
56) Country:
57) Name of partnership program (if applicable):
58) Partner classification:
    - □ Public academic institution
    - □ Private academic institution
    - □ Nongovernmental organization
    - □ Other
59) Type of partnership:
    - □ Medical professional trainee program
    - □ Collaborative research
    - □ Health systems development/capacity building
    - □ Learning & practicum experience
    - □ Other
60) If "other" please specify the type of partnership:
61) Partnership duration:

62) Name of in-country representative:

63) E-mail of in-country representative:

64) Phone number of in-country representative:

65) Name of second in-country representative:

66) E-mail of second in-country representative:

67) Phone number of second in-country representative:

68) Please indicate if you would like to be personally recognized for your participation in the survey.

    □ Yes

    □ No

69) Please indicate if you or your representative would be willing to participate in a 30-minute telephone follow-up interview.

    □ Yes

    □ No

Thank You!

Appendix B. International Institution Survey

In this survey we are using the definition of Global Health published by *Koplan, et al., Lancet, 2009 Jun 6; 373(9679): 1993–5: ". . . global health is an area for study, research, and practice that places a priority on improving health and achieving equity in health for all people worldwide. Global health emphasises transnational health issues, determinants, and solutions; involves many disciplines within and beyond the health sciences and promotes interdisciplinary collaboration; and is a synthesis of population-based prevention with individual-level clinical care."*

In addition, we define partnerships as mutually beneficial collaborations among two or more entities who are acting cooperatively toward one or more specific shared goals related to global health.

General Information

What is your name?

What is the name of the institution where you are primarily based?

Select the type of institution (e.g., private academic institution, public academic institution, NGO, government agency, or other agency).

In what country or countries does this institution operate?

What is your title or position?

Do you have a specific responsibility for global health at your institution?

If so, what is that responsibility?

What is your e-mail address?

What is your phone number?

1. If you represent an academic institution, which of the following degrees and programs with a focus on global health are offered by your own academic institution? Check all that apply.

One or more global health courses	
Certificate	
Undergraduate minor	
Undergraduate major	
Dual or joint undergraduate major	
MPH with global health concentration or track	
Masters (non-MPH) with global health concentration	
Doctoral (e.g., PhD, DrPH, etc.) with global health concentration	
Joint PhD with global health concentration	
Health professional (e.g., nursing, vet, medical) with global health concentration	
Postgraduate (e.g., fellowships, residency) with global health concentration	
Dual or joint graduate degree including global health	
Joint degree offered by a high-income country	
Other (free text)	

2. If you represent an academic institution, what are the health-related education and training programs your academic institution needs to augment?

3. Approximately how many global health partnerships does your institution have with universities in the following countries and/or regions:

Country/region	*Number of partnerships*
United States	
Canada	
Europe	
Latin America & Caribbean	
Africa	
Asia Pacific	
Other:____________	

4. What are the key focus areas of your global health partnerships with universities in the following countries and/or regions? Check all that apply.

	Not a focus area	*United States*	*Canada*	*Europe*	*Latin America & Caribbean*	*Africa*	*Asia Pacific*	*Other*
Medical professional education & training program								
Public health education & training program								
Collaborative research								
Development or delivery of interventions & services								
Health systems development/ capacity building								
Technology exchange								
Policy development & advocacy								
Learning & practicum experience for North American students								
Learning & practicum experience for your own students								
Maximizing global health impact								
Other (specify): ______________								

Comments:

5. On a scale of 1 to 5, please evaluate the overall strength and value-added of the partnerships that your institution has with the academic institutions listed below.

	No such partnership 0	*Poor* 1	*Fair* 2	*Good* 3	*Very good* 4	*Excellent* 5
North American partner universities						
European partner universities						
Latin American & Caribbean partner universities						
Asia-Pacific partner universities						
African partner universities						
Other (specify): ________						

Comments:

6. Overall, which of the following global health partnerships have been most valuable to you so far?

   - ☐ South-North partnerships
   - ☐ South-South partnerships

7. Which type of partnership will be your highest priority to develop in the future?

   - ☐ South-North partnerships
   - ☐ South-South partnerships

8. On a scale of 1 to 5, rate the extent to which the following areas are priorities for your institution's global health partnerships.

	Not a priority 1	*Low priority* 2	*Medium priority* 3	*High priority* 4	*Highest priority* 5
Knowledge acquisition for students					
Knowledge acquisition for faculty & administrators					

(continued)

	Not a priority 1	*Low priority 2*	*Medium priority 3*	*High priority 4*	*Highest priority 5*
Financial support					
Research support					
Health systems strengthening support					
Interventions or services implementation support					
Technology & equipment transfer					
Reciprocal student exchanges					
Maximizing global health impact					
Other (specify): ______					

Comments:

9. On a scale of 1 to 5, please indicate the degree of importance of different sources of North American funding and other funding that have been particularly critical for the success of your partnerships with North American academic institutions.

	Do not receive 0	*Not important 1*	*Low importance 2*	*Medium importance 3*	*High importance 4*	*Essential 5*
Your North American academic partner(s)						
International research agencies (e.g., NIH, Fogarty, Canadian IDRC, other—please specify)						
PEPFAR						
Medical Education Partnership Initiative (MEPI)						

	Do not receive 0	*Not important 1*	*Low importance 2*	*Medium importance 3*	*High importance 4*	*Essential 5*
Other North American government funding (e.g., CDC, USAID, CIDA, etc.)						
Nonfederal government funding/other external grants or contracts						
UN Agencies (e.g., WHO, UNAIDS, UNICEF, World Bank)						
International nongovernmental organizations						
Private donors						
Foundations (e.g., Gates, Rockefeller, Clinton)						
Private philanthropy						
Other (specify): ______						

Comments:

10. On a scale of 1 to 5, for your institution's partnership with a North American university that you know the most about, please indicate the extent to which the partnership is beneficial for your institution in the following areas.

	Not applicable *0*	*Harmful* *1*	*Not beneficial* *2*	*Somewhat beneficial* *3*	*Beneficial* *4*	*Very beneficial* *5*
Knowledge acquisition for students						
Knowledge acquisition for faculty & administrators						
Financial support						
Research support						
Health systems strengthening support						
Interventions or services implementation support						
Technology & equipment transfer						
Reciprocal student exchanges						
Maximizing global health impact						

Comments:

11. What health-related skill sets are most needed in your country and how can North American institutions help to develop and retain these skill sets?

12. What are the primary types of collaborations and investments that your institution receives from its university partners in the United States and/or Canada? Please describe what is supported by these investments.

	Y/N	*Provide specific examples of how each type of investment is utilized by your institution*
1. Cash resources		
2. Collaborative research grants		
3. Our students receive training		
4. Students and trainees from the North American partners help with education, research, or service at our institution		
5. Provision of advisers for our faculty		
6. North American academic support for Global Health educational curriculum development and/or delivery		
7. Other (specify): ______________		

13. On a scale of 1 to 5, rate the extent to which your institution's expectations are being met with regards to the overall adequacy and usefulness of collaborative investments received from your North American partners?

Does not meet your expectations 1	*Below your expectations 2*	*Meets some of your expectations 3*	*Meets all your expectations 4*	*Exceeds your expectations 5*

14. What have been the administrative and/or operational barriers, if any, to the success of your partnership(s) (e.g., MOUs, legal registration, visas, taxation policy, or other policies)?

15. Beyond financial and administrative support, what are the **top two or three** types of innovative support that your North American partners could provide that would be most useful in strengthening the impact of your partnerships on global health (e.g., joint courses or degrees, distance learning, assistance in grant writing, fellowships, mentoring of faculty, policy development, implementation science, etc.)?

Partnership Management

16. On a scale of 1 to 5, for the following categories, how adequate is the preparation of **North American** students hosted by your institution?

	Very inadequate 1	*Somewhat inadequate* 2	*Somewhat adequate* 3	*Adequate* 4	*Very adequate* 5
Ethical practices and our country's institutional requirements					
Sociocultural aspects of life in our country					
Cultural awareness for engaging in health work in low- and middle-income countries					
Language training					
Understanding of role, scope of tasks and supervision while in our country					
Prepared for the challenges of providing care or working in under-resourced settings					

Comments on preparation of North American students or trainees:

17. What kind of preparation is most important for North American students participating in global health projects and what can North American universities do to better prepare students participating in global health partnerships?

Evaluating Success

18. On a scale of 1 to 5, please rate how well your institution is working together with its North American partner universities in the following areas.

	Not done	*Poor* *1*	*Fair* *2*	*Well* *3*	*Very well* *4*	*Excellent* *5*
Assessing your institution's needs						
Establishing mutual goals						
Addressing the needs of your institution						
Planning, monitoring & evaluating the impact of collaborations						
Systematically providing feedback to your North American university partners						

Comments:

19. For each type of partnership listed below in which your institution has engaged, describe what specific characteristics and critical factors were necessary to make it **successful?**

Medical professional trainee program (e.g., medicine, nursing public health, pharmacy–please specify)	
Collaborative research	
Capacity building	
Learning and practicum experience for North American students	
Learning and practicum experience for your students	
Other (specify): ________________	

20. For each type of partnership listed below that your institution has engaged in, what are the specific factors that may have made it **less successful**?

Medical professional trainee program (e.g., medicine, nursing public health, pharmacy—please specify)	
Collaborative research	
Capacity building	
Learning and practicum experience for North American students	
Learning and practicum experience for your students	
Other (specify): ______________	

21. For the following categories, please rate on a scale of 1 to 5 how well your institution's needs are being met by your institution's **North American partners**.

	Not a focus area	*Poor 1*	*Fair 2*	*Well 3*	*Very well 4*	*Excellent 5*
Medical professional training program						
Collaborative research						
Clinical or public health interventions or services						
Health systems development/capacity building						
Technology exchange						
Policy development & advocacy						
Learning and practicum experience for students						
Other (specify): ______________						

Comments:

22. In your current partnerships with North American universities, what are the most important needs and interests that are not being adequately met by any of your partnerships and **what can be done to address what is lacking?**

23. What is the most exciting new opportunity for your institution's global health partnerships and how do you think your partnerships could jointly address this new opportunity?

24. In conclusion, can you identify specific areas of focus from the list below that your program is working on? Check all that apply.

__HIV/AIDS

__Malaria

__Tuberculosis

__Neglected tropical diseases

__Reproductive, maternal/neonatal, and child health

__Road traffic injuries

__Chronic noncommunicable diseases

__Development of policies that address tobacco and alcohol

__Health systems

__Air pollution

__Violence

__Mental health

__Other: Please enter an 'other' value for this selection

Thank you for your time

Please indicate if you would like to be personally recognized for your participation in the study. (You will not be linked to any specific responses).

Yes □ □ No

It will be extremely helpful to have a brief telephone conversation about topics presented in the surveys. Please indicate if you or another representative from your institution might be willing to participate in a 30-minute telephone follow-up interview to further discuss topics.

Yes □ □ No

Appendix C. Questions Posed During Interviews

1. Can you give a brief (e.g., five minute) overview of how your global health program was developed (e.g., when, how, why), including the role of international partnerships and details on how these partnerships have evolved over time?

2. Can you describe the importance and/or benefits of international partnerships for your global health program? Could you give an example of a partnership that highlights where these benefits have been realized?

3. Can you identify some of the key specific goals of your global health program and/or areas of focus that your institution is working on through its partnerships? (e.g., infectious diseases; HIV/AIDS, malaria; TB; neglected tropical diseases; reproductive, maternal neonatal and child health; road and traffic injuries; chronic noncommunicable diseases; development of policies that address tobacco, alcohol; health systems; development of new tools; air pollution; health economics research; etc.)

   And provide any concrete examples of specific outputs and/or outcomes from your international partnerships that support these goals?

4. What key factors have allowed your international partnerships to be successful?

5. What have been the challenges and what message would be valuable to spread to others so they could avoid the same pitfalls? Could you give an example of a partnership that highlights these challenges?

6. What are areas in which your partnerships could be improved and what would be needed to make these improvements?

7. What are key lessons learned from your global health program's experience with international partnerships that could be useful to others?

8. (Unstructured follow-up on any survey responses that require further exploration and/or clarification.)

9a. Scale of immediate sustainability (i.e., on a scale of 1 to 5, with 1 representing immediate termination and 5 representing highly sustainable and growing, how sustainable is your program currently?)

9b. Specific examples, what do you think will change in the near future?

9c. Five years from now, how do you think your program will have change?

10. With regards to your institution's global health program, what are the major current challenges and the major successes to date? (This is confidential.) Please provide concrete examples of specific outputs and/or outcomes.

11. What would be your top three suggestions to schools in the early stages of developing a global health program?

12. We're interested in how you conceptualize global health justice and equity. How do you define these concepts, and do you see them manifested in your program? If so, how?

Appendix D. List of North American Academic Institutions

Albert Einstein College of Medicine

Baylor College of Medicine

Boston University

Brown University

California Northstate University

Case Western Reserve University

Columbia University

Cornell University

Creighton University

Dalhousie University

Dartmouth University

DePaul University

Duke University

Emory University

Florida State University

George Washington University

Georgetown University

Harvard University

Indiana University

Johns Hopkins University

Long Island University

Loyola University Chicago

McGill University

McMaster University

Medical College of Wisconsin

Michigan State University

Morgan State University

Mount Sinai School of Medicine

New York University

North Carolina Central University

Northeastern University

Northwestern University

Ohio University

Rice University

Rosalind Franklin University of Medicine and Science

Rutgers University

San Diego State University

Stanford University

SUNY Downstate

SUNY Stony Brook

SUNY Upstate Medical University

Texas Tech University

Touro University

Tufts University

Tulane University

Uniformed Services University of the Health Sciences

University of Alabama at Birmingham

University of Alberta

University of Arizona

University of California, Berkeley

University of California, Los Angeles

University of California, San Diego

University of California, San Francisco

University of Chicago

University of Cincinnati

University of Denver

University of Illinois at Chicago

University of Iowa

University of Kentucky

University of Manitoba

University of Maryland, Baltimore

University of Maryland, College Park

University of Michigan

University of Minnesota

University of North Carolina

University of Notre Dame

University of Pennsylvania

University of Pittsburgh

University of Southern California

University of Texas

University of Toronto

University of Utah

University of Vermont

University of Virginia

University of Washington

University of Wisconsin–Madison

UT Southwestern Medical Center

Vanderbilt University

Washington State University

Washington University in St. Louis

West Virginia University

Yale University

Yeshiva University

Appendix E. List of International Partner Institutions

Armed Forces Medical College (AFMC), Pune, India

Ben Gurion University of the Negev

Bugando Medical Center

Centro de Estudos em Tabaco e Saúde, Escola Nacional de Saúde Pública, Fiocruz

Centro de Investigación y Docencia Económicas A.C. (CIDE)

Centro Medico Humberto Parra

CES University

Chiang Mai University

China University of Political Science and Law

Cinterandes Foundation

Debre Berhan University

Escuela Superior Politecnica del Litoral

Family Support Link (FASUL)

Friends in Global Health

Instituto Dominicano de Desarrollo Integral. Inc/Paraiso Assistance Program

International Centre for Diarrhoeal Disease Research, Bangladesh (icddr,b)

Jimma University (North American institution A partner)

Jimma University (North American institution B partner)

Karnataka Health Promotion Trust (KHPT)

Kazan State Medical University

Kenyatta National Hospital

Kilimanjaro Christian Medical Centre

Mahidol University

Makerere University (North American institution A partner)

Makerere University (North American institution B partner)

Mision Para Cristo/Iglesia del Cristo

Moi University

Nelson Mandela African Institution of Science and Technology

New Concept Information Systems

Papua New Guinea Institute of Medical Research

Partners for Health and Development in Africa (PHDA)

Peking University Health Science Center

Pontificia Universidad Católica del Ecuador

Sao Paulo University Medical School

ShiratiI KMT Hospital

Stellenbosch University

Universidad Nacional Pedro Henriquez Ureña

Universidad Peruana Cayetano Heredia

University of Dakar

University of Guyana

University of Malawi, The Polytechnic

University of Ruhuna

University of Rwanda (North American institution A partner)

University of Rwanda (North American institution B partner)

University of the Philippines, Manila

University of Zambia

University of Zimbabwe

Appendix F. Case Study Articles

Anandaraja (2008)	The Design and Implementation of a Multidisciplinary Global Health Residency Track at the Mount Sinai School of Medicine	Mount Sinai School of Medicine
Debas (2011)	The University of California Global Health Institute Opportunities and Challenges	University of California system
Francis (2012)	The Global Health Curriculum of Weill Cornell Medical College: How One School Developed a Global Health Program	Weill Cornell Medical College
Haq (2008)	Creating a Center for Global Health at the University of Wisconsin–Madison	University of Wisconsin–Madison
Koplan (2008)	The Emory Global Health Institute: Developing Partnerships to Improve Health Through Research, Training, and Service	Emory University
Landrigan (2011)[1]	New Academic Partnerships in Global Health: Innovations at Mount Sinai School of Medicine	Mount Sinai School of Medicine
Lorntz (2008)[2]	A Trans-University Center for Global Health	University of Virginia
Macfarlane (2008)	Think Globally, Act Locally, and Collaborate Internationally: Global Health Sciences at the University of California, San Francisco	University of California, San Francisco
Ozgediz (2008)	Surgical Training and Global Health Initial Results of a 5-Year Partnership with a Surgical Training Program in a Low-Income Country	University of California, San Francisco
Pinto (2014)	A case study of global health at the university: implications for research and action	University of Toronto
Quinn (2008)	The Johns Hopkins Center for Global Health: Transcending Borders for World Health	Johns Hopkins University
Saba (2008)	Beyond Borders: Building Global Health Programs at McGill University Faculty of Medicine	McGill University
Stapleton (2006)	Addressing Global Health Through the Marriage of Public Health and Medicine: Developing the University of Washington Department of Global Health	University of Washington

Vermund (2008)	Building Global Health Through a Center-Without-Walls: The Vanderbilt Institute for Global Health	Vanderbilt University
Watterson (2015)[3]	Building a Framework for Global Health Learning: An Analysis of Global Health Concentrations in Canadian Medical Schools	Canadian universities

1. P. J. Landrigan, J. Ripp, R. J. Murphy, L. Claudio, J. Jao, B. Hexom, H. G. Bloom, T. Shirazian, E. Elahi, and J. P. Koplan, "New Academic Partnerships in Global Health: Innovations at Mount Sinai School of Medicine," *Mount Sinai Journal of Medicine* 78, no. 3 (2011): 470–482
2. B. Lorntz, J. R. Boissevain, R. Dillingham, J. Kelly, A. Ballard, W. M. Scheld, and R. L. Guerrant, "A Trans-University Center for Global Health," *Academic Medicine* 83, no. 2 (2008): 165–172.
3. R. Watterson, D. Matthews, P. Bach, I. Kherani, M. Halpine, and R. Meili, "Building a Framework for Global Health Learning: An Analysis of Global Health Concentrations in Canadian Medical Schools," *Academic Medicine* 90, no. 4 (2015): 500–504.

About the Authors

Jonathan A. Muir is a PhD student in the Department of Sociology, an MPH student in the Department of Epidemiology, and is a START Research Assistant at the University of Washington. His research interests center on child and maternal health in Southeast Asia and sub-Saharan Africa, where he investigates the impact of armed conflict, trauma, and spatial inequality on child mortality and stunting. He has over 10 years of international research experience, primarily working with the peoples of Cambodia, Laos, Malaysia, Thailand, and Vietnam. As an avid linguist, he is fluent in Thai, conversant in Laotian, and currently studying Bahasa Indonesian and Khmer. His prior experience also includes working with refugees and victims of human trafficking.

Jessica Farley is an MPH student and START Research Assistant in the Department of Global Health at the University of Washington. After graduating with a BA degree in sociology/environmental studies from Whitman College, she spent three years living in West Africa as a Peace Corps volunteer, first in Mauritania integrating environmental education at the primary-school level, and later in Mali implementing health and forestry activities with community groups. Most recently, she worked for the global health organization PATH on an HIV-prevention project focused on key populations in low-income countries. Her interests include operations research, climate change adaptation within health systems, and HIV prevention.

Allison Osterman is a master's student in the Department of Global Health in the Health Metrics and Evaluation track at the University of Washington and a START Research Assistant. She received her BA in international studies from the University of Denver and earned a Professional Certificate in International Development from American University. Prior to joining UW, she worked as a monitoring and evaluation officer for the UN World Food Programme in Niger. She also worked as a program officer for the U.S. Agency for International Development in the Office of Food for Peace. While at USAID, she served as a food security focal point for the humanitarian response to the 2010 earthquake in Haiti.

Stephen E. Hawes, PhD, is an associate professor in the Department of Epidemiology and has adjunct appointments in the Departments of Global Health and Health Services at the University of Washington. He is the associate director of the Strategic Analysis and Research Training (START) Center, housed in the Department of Global Health. Dr. Hawes's primary research interests are in human papillomavirus (HPV) and human immunodeficiency virus (HIV). His current research projects are being conducted in Seattle and in Senegal,

West Africa, and concern the role of HIV, HPV, and other sexually transmitted infections in the natural history of cervical neoplasia and cancer. He also is involved in studies of biomarkers for various cancers and is a core faculty member at the UW Center for Excellence in Maternal and Child Health. Dr. Hawes teaches a number of courses in epidemiologic methods to undergraduate and graduate students.

Hon. Keith Martin, MD, PC, is a physician who, since September 2012, has served as the founding executive director of the Consortium of Universities for Global Health, based in Washington, D.C. Between 1993 and 2011, Dr. Martin served as a member of Parliament in Canada's House of Commons representing a riding on Vancouver Island. During that time, he held shadow ministerial portfolios in foreign affairs, international development, and health. He also served as Canada's parliamentary secretary for defense. In 2004, he was appointed to the Queen's Privy Council for Canada. His main areas of focus are in global health, foreign policy, security, international development, conservation, and the environment. Dr. Martin has been on numerous diplomatic missions to areas in crisis. He served as a physician in South Africa on the Mozambique border during that country's civil war. He has traveled widely in Africa, visiting the continent 26 times. He is the author of more than 150 published editorial pieces and has appeared frequently as a political and social commentator on television and radio. He is a board member of the Jane Goodall Institute, editorial board member for the *Annals of Global Health*, and an adviser for the International Cancer Expert Corps. He has contributed to the Lancet Commission on the Global Surgery Deficit; is a current commissioner on the Lancet-Icahn School of Medicine at Mount Sinai Commission on Pollution, Health and Development; and is a member of the Global Sepsis Alliance.

J. Stephen Morrison, PhD, is senior vice president at the Center for Strategic and International Studies in Washington, D.C., and director of its Global Health Policy Center. Dr. Morrison writes widely, has directed several high-level commissions, and is a frequent commentator on U.S. foreign policy, global health, Africa, and foreign assistance. He served in the administration of President Bill Clinton, as committee staff in the House of Representatives, and taught for 12 years at the Johns Hopkins School of Advanced International Studies. He holds a PhD in political science from the University of Wisconsin and is a magna cum laude graduate of Yale College.

King K. Holmes, MD, PhD, is professor of global health and medicine and adjunct professor of microbiology and epidemiology at the University of Washington. He is principal investigator for the UW/Fred Hutch Center for AIDS Research and for the International Training and Education Center for Health (I-TECH), a UW/UCSF collaboration with programs in 20 countries. He has collaborated with over 150 trainees and mentees on STI/HIV research and on over 750 publications, including 30 books and monographs. He is a member of the American Society for Clinical Investigation and the National Academy of Medicine and received the 2013 Canada Gairdner Foundation Global Health Award and the 2013 Infectious Diseases Society of America Lifetime Achievement Award.

www.ingramcontent.com/pod-product-compliance
Ingram Content Group UK Ltd.
Pitfield, Milton Keynes, MK11 3LW, UK
UKHW051418150926
475561UK00005B/224

9 781442 259089